ALZHEIMER'S TREATMENTS

THAT ACTUALLY WORKED

IN SMALL STUDIES BUT

WILL NEVER BE TESTED &

YOU WILL NEVER HEAR ABOUT

FROM YOUR MD OR
BIG PHARMA

BECAUSE THEY ARE UNPATENTABLE,
UNPROFITABLE, AND EASILY OBTAINABLE!!

Jeff T. Bowles

This book is dedicated to

The pioneering research and theoretical works of

Dr. Vladimir Dilman and Dr. Ward Dean.

Introduction

I apologize for not writing this book 15 years ago in 1997, when I first developed a novel, compelling theory about the cause of and potential treatments for Alzheimer's disease. Why did I sit on this information for so long? Let me explain by giving you a little of its history.

I personally have seen the toll that Alzheimer's can take on a great mind. My grandfather got the disease in his 60's, when he was a very well-respected lawyer/real estate investor/ politician. When it first hit him, we noticed he would keep driving with the turn indicator on. After he was diagnosed, we noticed his vocabulary started a rapid decline, when he would look out the window and talk about the birds he would like to feed, and would refer to them as tails. He would drive my grandmother crazy by getting up at night and being all agitated. They finally sent him to a nursing home. I remember that when I went to visit him (when I was 14), he would just sit in a wheel chair and could not hold his head up, could not speak, and would drool a lot. He looked terrible! He died of pneumonia not too long after I saw him like that. They probably decided not to treat him.

1997 was the year when I was the first who theorized that the dramatic increases of human *Luteinizing Hormone* (LH) that occurs in aging people (by up to 1,000's of percent) is the culprit that causes Alzheimer's disease.

At the time, this was quite a radical idea that had never been seen before in print or even mentioned by anyone, sane or insane! You see, *Luteinizing Hormone* (LH) was supposed to be a hormone that only affected, controlled, and acted upon sex-related tissues.

By June, 1997, I had finished a theoretical paper describing this crazy idea, and it was accepted for publication by the British journal, *Medical Hypotheses*, and eventually made it into print in September, 1998. The theory was still quite speculative at the time, but little by little, supporting facts started trickling in.

About a year after my paper was published, LH receptors were found all over the body (and in the brain), not just in the sex tissues. About a year after that, the Mayo clinic found that autopsied brains of Alzheimer's victims were *loaded* with LH, with the heaviest concentrations being found in the *most damaged parts of the brain.*

Just last year, a paper by a scientist at the NIH (the conservative US government-run National Institutes of Health) agreed that he (and they) *now* believe the premise is correct--that LH *does* cause Alzheimer's! Quite a turnaround from the initial ridicule I got from various Alzheimer's researchers to whom I'd mentioned the LH idea.

I remember one researcher from Northwestern University, standing in front of his highly complicated amyloid beta poster, telling me, "I wish it were that easy," and then smugly turning his back on me. But that is typical behavior when you are proposing unfamiliar ideas to most scientists. In my experience, I have not found much difference in my dealings with scientists and with autistic children.

How are scientists like autistic children? They both usually share these characteristics:

- they are socially awkward
- they have and concentrate intensely on *peculiar interests*
- they are usually pedantic (enjoy correcting others and demonstrating their detailed knowledge of a topic)
- they love repetition and *sameness* (thus, they're not particularly creative)
- and, they get *really* upset when the furniture is rearranged!

Another researcher, after reading my paper at my suggestion, said that even though he wasn't exactly sure about all the ideas presented in it, his initial opinion was that if it was a painting instead of a science article, it seemed more like something his granddaughter might have created, as opposed to a Jackson Pollock. Several times I got letters back from well-known, evolution professors that started with something like, "Unfortunately you do not understand how evolution works."

It used to make me angry, and I would go into a tirade showing them how wrong they were--but now it just makes me laugh. The mainstream science community cannot be convinced of anything new, no matter how much proof you push into their faces. That is why I no longer write papers for scientists--only for those who might be able to fairly evaluate the facts and theories I present. Today's mainstream professional scientists will be the last to accept any changes to their beliefs. It really is a sad situation, because it leads to a snail's pace of scientific and medical advancement on which countless suffering humans are waiting. In this book, I will discuss how the entire medical, evolutionary, biology, and science communities are all trapped in a self-policed and self-reinforced logical box which prevents them from coming up with proper, simple, approaches for treating the diseases of aging which today would be considered "outside the box." I will also explain how to get *out of the box* without violating the rules of logic.

Chapter 1. Foundations of the Theory

When I submitted my first paper (a unified theory of aging) to the journal, *Experimental Gerontology,* the Editor-in-Chief was Leonard Hayflick, a paragon in gerontology. Dr. Hayflick sent me a 3-page hand-written rejection letter, explaining to me that I did not know the first thing about aging. Leonard Hayflick is famous for discovering that human cells can undergo a finite number of replications before becoming senescent and unable to divide anymore. This is now called *the Hayflick limit.* Before Leonard came along, everyone thought cells could divide forever. But it turned out that the scientists keeping cell cultures alive were feeding them with chicken serum which contained *live* cells, which kept the culture "alive." Leonard corrected this erroneous belief, and became famous. He is now immortalized in history as the discoverer of the finite number of replications of a eukaryotic cell, this number forever being known as the "Hayflick Limit." Congratulations, Leonard. You solved the chicken serum problem! (Actually, he's an OK guy, and means well).

What is LH?

Luteinizing hormone (LH) is a huge hormone. One molecule of it weighs 28,000 grams per mole, while testosterone weighs just 288 grams per mole. (What is a mole? It is the number of molecules (atoms in this case) in 12 grams of Carbon (randomly chosen by early scientists as a standard unit). So LH is 100 times bigger/heavier than a molecule of testosterone--or estrogen, for that matter--and about 1,400 times bigger than an atom of Carbon! It consists of 2 halves--the *alpha* unit and the *beta* unit, about equal in size. The only thing unique about the LH hormone is the *beta* unit. The LH alpha unit is identical to the alpha unit in the other large hormone molecules, FSH (follicle stimulating hormone), TSH (thyroid stimulating hormone) and hCG (human chorionic gonadotropin) (One might guess that the larger the hormone molecule, the older it is, from an evolutionary point of view, because as the hormone molecule gets bigger, the receptor has to get bigger--and that should take time). Anyway, this is too much information! Let's get back to what matters--the simple stuff.

The conventional view is that in women, a monthly surge in LH drives the dissolution of the egg-containing follicle by triggering the production of prostaglandins and proteolytic enzymes that weaken the follicle's wall. A follicle is basically a pimple with an egg inside that starts to get bigger and eventually pops. (LH also stimulates the remnants of the burst follicle to become a little hormone-producing gland called "the corpus luteum" which secretes various hormones after the follicle has ruptured [including lots of progesterone--this will be important later]). After the follicle bursts, the ovum (egg) is released into the Fallopian tube where it can become fertilized. The important function of LH for our purposes is that it initially drives the destruction of tissue in this process.

In men, LH stimulates the testes to secrete testosterone, and is central to promoting fertility and sperm production in males. (I'm guessing that it eats away the tissue housing the developing sperm, and allows it to be released--but I don't know for sure, as I haven't researched it. But I'm guessing this function of LH [if it exists] probably won't be discovered for a while). LH increases are also involved in triggering and driving puberty in both juvenile males and females.

How did I come up with such a crazy idea that a sex-related hormone that was good for you when you were younger and only acted on your sex tissues somehow became a killer that attacked your brain when you got older? It all began with my writing a paper that summed up 15 years of independent research that I had been doing, regarding the evolutionary purpose and biochemical/hormonal basis of aging in humans. (And I mean *really* independent! I worked for no one but myself. My goal was to answer the riddle of aging. I did it for free, for sometimes 12 hours a day when I was on a hot lead, and often 7 days a week--for years).

I had been working on my own for years on learning everything about aging I could get my hands on, from any source possible, and had been refining a unified theory of aging. In early 1997, I finally was able to lay most of the hormonal blame for human aging on two sex-related hormones--FSH (follicle stimulating hormone) and LH (luteinizing hormone). These hormones both increase dramatically after age 40 in both men and women (and become much more immuno- and bio-active and take longer to dissipate). But I must give the bulk of the credit to "my discovery" to a book I read many times--The Neuroendocrine Theory of Aging and Degenerative Disease, by Vladimir Dilman and Ward Dean. Even though I think the cover looks somewhat unscientific, this book is definitely a good resource--a true case of "don't judge a book by its cover!" The Neuroendocrine Theory had charts showing changes in various hormone levels in people over their lifetimes--and the evidence was right there--HUGE increases in LH and FSH after age 40 in both men and women. Dilman and Dean explained that the rise in LH and FSH were due to a loss of sensitivity to negative feedback inhibition by hormones-a process which is responsible for both development and aging. Changes in hormone receptor sensitivity are responsible for the long term increases in various hormones throughout life, which ultimately results

13

in hormonal conditions that lead to most of the diseases of aging which <u>they identified</u> as obesity, hypertension, diabetes, cardiovascular disease, immune dysfunction, depression, and cancer.

(I happen to have a somewhat different list of aging-related diseases that <u>does not</u> include obesity, hypertension, depression, or diabetes and relegates them to a syndrome associated with Vitamin D3 deficiency (lack of sun) which I call the human hibernation syndrome and discuss at length in a book I wrote about Vitamin D3. Time will tell which version of the hormonal theory of aging is the most correct.)

Given that these "hibernation" diseases of depression, hypertension, diabetes, and obesity were primarily seen in older, aging adults when Dilman devised his theory, adding them to the aging category was certainly logical. However since the first publication of Dilman's theory in 1955, the US population has undergone a huge experiment in mass Vitamin D3 deficiency beginning in the 1980's when doctors started warning everyone to avoid the sun and use sunscreen. Since then we have seen obesity, hypertension, and even type 2 diabetes skyrocket in children-thus providing one leg of the logic to remove them from the general diseases of aging category.

(Heart disease might also be a sub-part of the human hibernation syndrome (related to seasonal variations of Vitamin K2 in the diet-K2 levels are high in vegetation in the summer and low or nonexistent in the winter) but I am not quite ready to banish heart disease from the list of aging-related diseases just yet. Maybe heart disease belongs in both categories- I am still working on this idea.)

In all fairness to Drs. Dean and Dilman, one could make the case that the human hibernation syndrome /Vitamin D3 deficiency theory could be merged with the hormonal theory of aging given that as one ages the ability of one's skin to make Vitamin D3 from sunlight declines dramatically. Thus, one might be justified in saying that age-related Vitamin D3 deficiency was part of the overall aging process...Back to the main argument-

Their theory explained that the "good" hormones decline with age, which I believe is the major part of the correct hormonal theory of aging-why? Because declines in some "good" hormones like melatonin lead to increases in other "bad" hormones like LH and FSH-(more on this later). Although Dilman had all of the important facts right, he missed one major aspect that would have properly completed his theory, with regard to Alzheimer's disease, osteoporosis and a number of other conditions associated with aging that involve atrophy of somatic tissues such as hearing and vision loss, sarcopenia (muscle wasting) , arthritis, joint destruction, dementia, etc. . Dilman and Dean had the evidence to properly complete their theory- that LH and FSH were "bad" pro-aging hormones, right before their eyes, –they just didn't see it! Here's a little graph from a study of LH and FSH levels based on age:

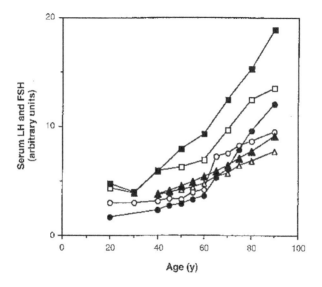

In addition to the huge rise in LH and FSH, hCG goes way up in men and women after age 40 (and is very similar structurally to LH). As far as reproduction is concerned, hCG (human Chorionic Gonadotropin) causes the woman's uterus to prepare for and maintain egg implantation. Without it, there would be no pregnancy. Unknown to some scientists (like one I talked to from the Dana Farber Cancer Center, at Harvard) men also make hCG. I bet him at a conference dinner that men produced hCG. He said "no way. *I'm* from the Dana Farber Cancer Center," he boasted. Well, he lost the bet. He was mortified since *he* was the so-called *expert*. hCG is almost identical to LH, and can attach to LH receptors. In fact, they are called LH-CG receptors.

I finally found one obscure study that showed, as I expected, men and women's hCG levels increase dramatically after age 40 by about 500%, on average. This should be of concern to those who use hCG for dieting purposes, and athletes who use it to boost their testosterone production (i.e. Manny Ramirez, who was suspended from baseball for 50 games for using it). Human chorionic gonadotropin also plays a role in cellular differentiation/proliferation and may activate apoptosis (aka, *cell suicide*).

I also found that human aging involved the dramatic-decline of some so-called "good hormones" after age 40. DHEA, melatonin, pregnenolone, growth hormone, and progesterone (after age 70 in men, and after age 35 in women), as well as testosterone in men and women, and estrogen in women. Estrogen/estradiol has both good and bad effects on aging for both sexes, and is a cAMP-stimulating hormone (see below). The decline of Vitamin D3 (actually, a hormone, made when sun hits the skin) is also on the list of good hormones that decline with age. Why? Because as one gets older, the ability of one's skin to create Vitamin D3 declines dramatically.

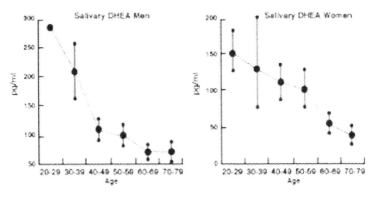

Fig. 2: Typical DHEA levels in men and women.

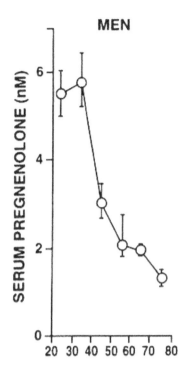
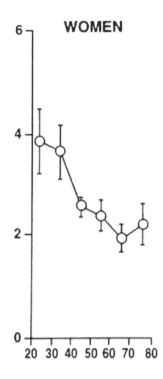

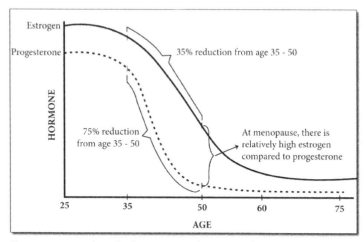

Progesterone levels in women by age-There are no charts that I could find for men.

(For those of you who are interested in more advanced biochemical ideas, I found that all the "good" hormones bind to receptors which then stimulate the release of cyclic GMP (cGMP) while all the "bad" ones generally stimulate receptors which then cause the release of cyclic AMP (cAMP). I also found that when cruising the Pub Med database, if you type in each of the cGMP-stimulating hormones vs. cancer, you find almost *no evidence* of cGMP-stimulating hormones involved in promoting cancers, while almost every cAMP stimulating hormone (except FSH) is associated with various cancers. cGMP and cAMP are known as second messengers. When a hormone hits a hormone receptor on a cell, it triggers the 2nd message that actually tells the DNA what to do. Also, the A in cAMP is the same A in the GCAT of DNA, and the same with the G in cGMP. I also theorized in my paper that the cGMP pathway is the antioxidant signaling pathway, while the cAMP is the free radical signaling pathway).

While researching luteinizing hormone (LH) in 1997, I stumbled across two interesting studies. One suggested that cigarette smoking caused a drop in LH. The other study showed that Ibuprofen also led to LH decreases in chronic users. This was my "eureka" moment, because I had also seen studies that linked cigarette smoking and Ibuprofen use to *lower incidence of Alzheimer's disease*! I finished my theory paper with a section on how LH likely caused Alzheimer's disease.

To the contrary, there are also a few other studies out there that suggest that heavy smoking in middle age in Finlanders actually *increases* the risk of Alzheimer's, which got a lot of press. *Nothing* seems completely simple when you are trying to ascribe a single effect to a single hormone in a somewhat diverse population such as humans. It is possible that Finlanders have low Vitamin D3 levels due to lack of sun, which, combined with smoking, may lead to AD. There are many confounding variables, so it's best not to get hung up on single "outlier" studies if you don't have to. Anyway, the vast majority of studies suggest that smoking *prevents* Alzheimer's as well as Parkinson's disease.

The section on how LH might cause Alzheimer's was in my paper, "The Evolution of Aging: A New Approach to an Old Problem of Biology," and it was published in September, 1998 by the British journal, *"Medical Hypotheses."*

1998 would have been about the earliest I could have written a book on Alzheimer's. However, I did not have enough confidence that my theory was correct to warrant such an undertaking. Also, back in 1997-8 it was quite difficult to publish a book, as one had to find a publisher willing to take a gamble on an unknown author.

The invention of e-book publishing has changed that equation totally, and allowed me to get this important message out to you quickly, efficiently, and cheaply. So why didn't I write this book anywhere from 2000 until now? That's a whole different story, which I will get into later. But for now, I can say I was waiting for our science community and Big Pharma to take the ball and run with it. Instead, the ball was *horribly fumbled*, and remains so-- more on this later.

Chapter Two—Lupron for Alzheimer's disease.

The Story behind the Story.

I will take a break in laying out all the facts and theory leading up to the most promising treatment for Alzheimer's known to mankind and its history--and tell you the most likely *best treatments for Alzheimer's* based on my research right now. Then we can return to laying out the facts, theory, and evidence to get the total story.

The bottom line facts are that:

1. The evidence that LH causes Alzheimer's disease has grown dramatically since 1998.

2. The most promising treatment for AD should be to *suppress LH!*

With this information you should have all the information you need to stop Alzheimer's in its tracks. However, there is a slight problem with this approach.

A small study showed that suppressing LH stops Alzheimer's from progressing in women, but *not* in men. In this study, *both* the experimental group and the control group received the commonly-prescribed drugs for

Alzheimer's disease--acetyl-cholinesterase inhibitors such as Aricept, Razadyne, Exelon or Cognex. The control group, which *did* decline, *only* got the acetyl-cholinesterase inhibitors, while the experimental group that *did not decline* got acetyl-cholinesterase inhibitors *plus* high-dose *Lupron* (aka Leuprolide Acetate)—a synthetic gonadotropin inhibitor, which suppresses LH.

Is this really true? Has suppressing LH ever been shown to stop the progression of AD in women? If you ask most scientists in the Alzheimer's field, or anyone associated with Big Pharma, they will answer, No--there is no treatment ever devised that has stopped Alzheimer's in its tracks in anyone, male or female.

However, they don't know about or don't trust the results of the one small Phase II trial in women just mentioned, where AD appeared to be completely stopped. So the happy answer to this question is, *YES--LH suppression has stopped AD in women.* This is still unknown to most in the AD industry, because it was done by scientists who I call "the gang who couldn't shoot straight," aka Voyager Pharmaceuticals. They were easily dismissed by our semi-autistic scientists who don't like the furniture getting rearranged.

The small study I just mentioned is a completely under- or

even un-reported study that showed that suppressing LH in women over 6 months with an off-the-shelf drug, leuprolide acetate (brand name *Lupron*), *totally* halted the decline in about 54 women with mild AD. The women were given the drug in a Phase II trial financed/run by a small start-up called *Voyager Pharmaceuticals*, in 2004. As mentioned, 54 women with AD who did not get Lupron injections continued to decline. Both groups were on traditional Alzheimer's drugs as well. Below is the graph they provided.

In this subgroup analysis, the mean ADAS-Cog score in the group receiving the high dose of leuprolide acetate and an ACI worsened by 0.18 points at week 48 from baseline compared to a mean worsening of 3.30 points in the group receiving placebo and an ACI. The p-value for this difference was 0.026 on an unadjusted basis and 0.078 on an adjusted basis. The following graph illustrates the results of this subgroup analysis of ADAS-Cog scores:

ALADDIN I-Phase II Trial
ADAS-Cog Scores (Intent-to-Treat Analysis)
ACI + High Dose Leuprolide Acetate versus ACI + Placebo

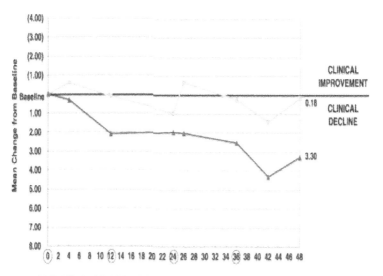

Visit Week (Dosing visit circled; patient assessment dates shown by squares and triangles)

ACI's + High Dose Leuprolide Acetate N [24] ＊ ACI's + Placebo N [26]

This was *huge* news to many, and it attracted Tommy Thompson, the ex-governor of Wisconsin, and ex-Health & Human Services Secretary of George Bush, and Michael Reagan (Ronald Reagan's son--the US's most famous Alzheimer's patient), as well as Sheldon Goldberg--once head of the US Alzheimer's Association, to all join the board of Voyager Pharmaceuticals. Talk of a Noble prize was in the air, and Voyager filed to raise $100 million from investors, with the same investment banker that took Google public. They had already burned through $50 million they had raised from a group of private investors. Everything was going great, until about a day before the IPO in late 2005, when the co-founder of Voyager and "discoverer" of the Lupron treatment for AD, Dr. Richard Bowen, had what many at the company called a nervous breakdown. A few months after their IPO was shelved, their Phase II study with Lupron for men with AD showed that Lupron DID NOT halt the progression of AD in men! OOPS!?

After the IPO was terminated, and Dr Bowen was kicked out of Voyager, it limped along and is almost dead, as we speak. Voyager recently changed its name to Curaxis, and fired all remnants of the old management to try to leave the controversies behind. It also did a reverse merger with a bankrupt (but listed) stock just to get listed. But as of today, Curaxis' stock trades for only 2 cents a share. I have $5,000 worth, if it ever comes back up to $1.50 again! How Voyager/Curaxis continues to screw me! You can read about the whole crazy affair by going to Yahoo Groups and typing in VYGR, which was to be their stock symbol. VYGR in Yahoo groups--now closed--was basically a "bitch and moan" group for all the Voyager investors who lost their $50 million of start-up money to the company's ineptitude and "bad luck" of initially discovering that Lupron stops Alzheimer's disease by monitoring the case of a MALE prostate cancer patient who had AD (supposedly, it doesn't work in men, remember!?).

Because Voyager did not invent Lupron, their only hope for making a profit was to get a use-patent on Lupron to treat Alzheimer's--which they did—but which would be kind of hard to enforce. A use-patent allows them to prevent others from using it to treat Alzheimer's. Like I said, hard to enforce--like getting a patent on air to prevent people from suffocating. Even though they have what seems to be the cure for AD in women, because they did not invent the drug, they will eventually find that it would be almost impossible for them to make a profit from it. Actually, Voyager *did* get a company called *Durect Pharmaceuticals* to create a Leuprolide Acetate implant that goes under one's skin and delivers a constant dose over several months, called *Memryte*. But other than that, they have no real protection to keep patients from buying and using generic Lupron, and not paying Voyager a royalty. Thus, the drug will likely never be studied again by Big Pharma, since it would be too hard to make any money from it. Lupron and similar drugs have been available for more than 20 years, and Lupron is scheduled to come off patent in 2015. Right now, it is quite expensive. It can be purchased cheaper in Canada for about $1,800 per year for the *regular* dose, but keep in mind that Voyager was using "high dose" Lupron injections for its Phase II study. Big Pharma could care less about your Alzheimer's disease if they cannot make money from it!

So--an excellent treatment for Alzheimer's in women exists which is not being made well-known to the public, because a small Pharma company is still trying, against all odds, to make a profit on it--and Big Pharma realizes it *cannot* make a profit from it! After Curaxis finally bites the dust, the great promise of using Lupron to stop Alzheimer's in women will simply fade away unless we, the stupid, sheep-like masses of guinea pigs for Big Pharma, make a stand and do the studies ourselves!

Here are the side effects of Lupron I found on the internet. I suggest you try high-dose melatonin, pregnenolone, DHEA and progesterone, *before* you try Lupron. (More on these treatments later in the book)

Side Effects of Lupron - for the Consumer (from drugs.com)

Lupron

All medicines may cause side effects, but many people have no, or minor, side effects. Check with your doctor if any of these most COMMON side effects persist or become bothersome when using Lupron:

Constipation; dizziness; general body pain; headache; hot flashes; loss of appetite; nausea or vomiting; stuffy nose; trouble sleeping; weakness.

Seek medical attention right away if any of these SEVERE side effects occur when using Lupron:
Severe allergic reactions (rash; hives; itching; difficulty breathing; tightness in the chest; swelling of the mouth, face, lips, or tongue); black, tarry stools; blood in the urine; burning, numbness, tingling, or weakness; decreased hearing; fainting; fever; mood or mental changes (e.g., depression); new or worsening bone pain; paralysis; redness or hardening of the skin at the injection site; seizures; severe dizziness or light-headedness; severe drowsiness; severe headache; shortness of breath or cough; slow, fast, or irregular heartbeat; sweating; swelling of the hands, ankles, or feet; symptoms of heart attack (e.g., chest, jaw, or left arm pain; numbness of an arm or leg; sudden, severe headache or vomiting; vision changes); symptoms of high blood sugar (e.g., drowsiness; fast breathing; flushing; fruit-like breath odor; increased thirst, hunger, or urination); symptoms of stroke (e.g., confusion, one-sided weakness, slurred speech, vision changes); unusual bruising or bleeding; unusual stomach pain; urination problems (e.g., trouble urinating, inability to urinate, painful urination); vision changes or blurred vision; vomit that looks like coffee grounds; yellowing of the skin or eyes.

This is not a complete list of all side effects that may occur. If you have questions about side effects, contact your health care provider. Call your doctor for medical advice about side effects.

Chapter 3—Treatments for Alzheimer's
that Work for Men *and* Women

If you are a woman you may be somewhat relieved now-- you know of *one* treatment for AD that *should* work for you. But if you are a man, you are still anxious and wondering--what treatment is there for me?

I will not disappoint you. If you are a man, taking around 120 mg a day of **melatonin** at night when you go to bed should, I believe, stop AD in its tracks. It should also work in women, and will likely be *way cheaper* and more fun for them than the Lupron injections, which have significant side effects already described.

Is there any evidence that melatonin can stop AD in men? Happily, YES there is.

The evidence is scant right now, but it is the best hope you have. I am highly optimistic about it. Doctors observed two men with Alzheimer's in 1995, who both got Alzheimer's at about the same age. One started taking 6mg of melatonin at night for sleep, while the other didn't. After three years, the melatonin-taking AD patient had almost no progression at all with his disease. He remained at stage 5 on the FAST scale (see Appendix C, Alzheimer's Clinical Stages). Stage

5 means he needed help picking out his clothes to wear.

However, the other patient had a dramatic decline in his ability to function--barely able to understand single words. He declined to about the lowest level on the FAST scale--7b, where he could not even withhold his urine or stool, and was limited to a small vocabulary of single words and grunts, and could barely hold his head up.

You might think this evidence sounds flimsy. Just two patients, both get AD about the same age and same time, one takes melatonin and does not progress much, while the other does not take melatonin and declines dramatically.

Well, I can hear you thinking right now. You could chalk it up to all sorts of things like genetics, environment etc. This is certainly what Big Pharma and AD scientists would have done. But they, of course, intentionally overlooked one interesting fact:

These two patients were identical twins! A virtual 100% DNA copy of each other. And they both got AD at almost the same time! (see Appendix B—Two Twins with Alzheimer's).

I find the description of their cases extremely exciting, promising and compelling! Why? Because *melatonin suppresses LH*! And this jibes exactly with my theory and the evidence from the Phase II trial in women given Lupron injections. The only thing I can fault these doctor/researchers for is not trying even *higher* doses of melatonin. You see, 6 mg is not much at all. Doses of melatonin as high as 75 mg/night have been used successfully in women in Europe for birth control. So if 6 mg seems to work, 75 mg might work up to 10 times better. I would adjust the 75 mg for women to an even higher dose for men--maybe 120 mg per night, due to weight differences. In fact, I have taken much higher doses--up to 500 mg per night--over a one year period, with no serious side effects, which I will describe in detail later.

Now, what did Big Pharma think about this 1998 observation? Absolutely nothing. They would rather say, "Oh, it's only 2 patients--way too small a sample size--best to ignore it."

A real reason they could choose to ignore it is that there *are* differences, even between twins, and this could account for the different outcomes for the two cases of Alzheimer's diseases. However, if I or you had to put money on it, we would have to bet that melatonin was stopping AD in the one twin, and that it *wasn't* an effect of rare differences between identical twins. Anyway, the real reason that it is best for Big Pharma to ignore the twin study is because they cannot make any money from melatonin, which is an over-the-counter unpatentable hormone/supplement. One way they might try to crack this nut is to create a slightly different chemical isotope of melatonin that still retains its physiological effects, rename it, and then get the FDA to outlaw melatonin. And this is exactly what one scientist has been trying to do. It never amazes me as to how crooked, greedy, and corrupt the Big Pharma and science communities can be.

If you have been following this reasoning closely, you would be asking yourself, "Why would melatonin stop Alzheimer's in males by suppressing LH? Didn't we just learn that suppressing LH in men has no effect on the progression of AD?" Well, good for you! You are paying attention.

When Voyager got the results that suppressing LH in men had no effect on slowing the progression of AD, they were caught with their pants down. Why? Because their lead researcher, Dr. Richard Bowen, had supposedly discovered that Leuprolide Acetate (aka Lupron) stopped Alzheimer's disease by monitoring a *single* patient back in the 1990's. The patient was a male who had prostate cancer *and* Alzheimer's (which ran in his family). Dr. Bowen noticed that Lupron treatments for his prostate cancer *totally stopped the progression of his AD*. OOPS! One little problem-- In his later studies, Lupron only stopped AD in women.

Dr Bowen, who had previously run 10 diet pill Phen/Fen clinics in Florida, and was fighting bankruptcy in 1997, noticed something that 20,000 urologists treating prostate cancer worldwide over the prior 20 years had not noticed. Bowen noticed that Lupron treatment for prostate cancer also stopped Alzheimer's in men!

It seems as if Dr. Bowen was not being completely up front as to the inspiration for "his discovery." I might tell you more on this later.

The bottom line is--melatonin not only suppresses LH in both men and women, it also increases progesterone levels in women (and I am going to guess in men, also, since there are no readily available data that I could find). Why do I guess this? As you will soon see, my theories led me to believe that *increasing progesterone levels in men* will stop Alzheimer's--*not* *decreasing LH levels*. Thus, because melatonin seemed to stop AD in one of the twins with AD, I have to guess that melatonin, as it does in women, also *increases progesterone levels in men*. This part is still theoretical. It might be that melatonin alters the entire milieu of hormones in men to stop the progression of AD, and progesterone has nothing to do with it.

So for our purposes, we can assume that melatonin works to stop the progression of AD in men by unknown means. Theory suggests it might be a boost in progesterone levels, and if it works in women, it probably does so by suppressing LH--which we know works from the Voyager experiment. Melatonin should work in both men and women, and has fewer negative side effects than Lupron. I will detail the side effects of both high-dose melatonin and Lupron, later.

The only thing I *did* find that suggests that melatonin might increase progesterone in men is a study where they treated adrenal cells of dogs with melatonin (see Appendix A), and this increased their cells' output of progesterone. This is good enough for me for now. Why?

When Voyager had determined that suppressing LH in men did not halt AD, I started wondering, why not? It was a big surprise to me in 2006 when I learned that Voyager's study results appeared to indicate that Lupron didn't work for Alzheimer's disease in men. That was another big reason I did not write this book sooner.

All I know for sure right now is that high dose melatonin should work in men to stop Alzheimer's in its tracks, based on the twin study. But that's all I have right now, unless someone can prove that melatonin boosts progesterone in men. It is well known that melatonin boosts progesterone in women. Melatonin probably does this in men, also (we need a study on this, please!)--so I should explain to you why I think progesterone supplementation should also stop Alzheimer's in its tracks for men.

Before we move on, I want to add some new exciting information that came to me from a reader as I was working on some revisions to this book...

Recently, it was shown in a mouse model of Alzheimer's disease that melatonin supplementation plus daily exercise halted their AD in its tracks. The article follows:

Melatonin and Exercise Work against Alzheimer's In Mice

Spanish Foundation for Science and Technology

Different anti-aging treatments work together and add years of life

The combination of two neuroprotective therapies, voluntary physical exercise, and the daily intake of melatonin has been shown to have a synergistic effect against brain deterioration in rodents with three different mutations of Alzheimer's disease.

A study carried out by a group of researchers from the Barcelona Biomedical Research Institute (IIBB), in collaboration with the University of Granada and the Autonomous University of Barcelona, shows the combined effect of neuroprotective therapies against Alzheimer's in mice.

Daily voluntary exercise and daily intake of melatonin, both of which are known for the effects they have in regulating circadian rhythm, show a synergistic effect against brain deterioration in the 3xTg-AD mouse, which has three mutations of Alzheimer's disease.

"For years we have known that the combination of different anti-aging therapies such as physical exercise, a Mediterranean diet, and not smoking adds years to one's life," Coral Sanfeliu, from the IIBB, explains to SINC.

"Now it seems that melatonin, the sleep hormone, also has important anti-aging effects".

The experts analyzed the combined effect of sport and melatonin in 3xTg-AD mice which were experiencing an initial phase of Alzheimer's and presented learning difficulties and changes in behavior such as anxiety and apathy.

The mice were divided into one control group and three other groups which would undergo different treatments: exercise –unrestricted use of a running wheel–, melatonin –a dose equivalent to 10 mg per kg of body weight–, and a combination of melatonin and voluntary physical exercise. In addition, a reference group of mice were included which presented no mutations of the disease.

"After six months, the state of the mice undergoing treatment was closer to that of the mice with no mutations than to their own initial pathological state. From this we can say that the disease has significantly regressed," Sanfeliu states.

The results, which were published in the journal *Neurobiology of Aging*, show a general improvement in behavior, learning, and memory with the three treatments.

These procedures also protected the brain tissue from oxidative stress and provided good levels of protection from excesses of amyloid beta peptide and hyperphosphorylated TAU protein caused by the mutations. In the case of the mitochondria, the combined effect resulted in an increase in the analyzed indicators of improved performance which were not observed independently.

"Transferring treatments which are effective in animals to human patients is not always consistent,* given that in humans the disease develops over several years, so that when memory loss begins to surface, the brain is already very deteriorated," the IIBB expert points out.

However, several clinical studies have found signs of physical and mental benefits in sufferers of Alzheimer's resulting from both treatments. The authors maintain that, until an effective pharmacological treatment is found, adopting healthy living habits is essential for reducing the risk of the disease appearing, as well as reducing the severity of its effects.

*Treatment not easily transferable to humans" (My note--they _always_ say this! Wouldn't want to cut into drug sales, right!)

The melatonin debate

The use of melatonin, a hormone synthesized from the neurotransmitter serotonin, has positive effects which can be used for treating humans. With the approval of melatonin as a medication in the European Union in 2007, clinical testing on this molecule has been increasing. It has advocates as well as detractors, and the scientific evidence has not yet been able to unite the differing views.

According to the Natural Medicines Comprehensive Database, melatonin is probably effective in sleeping disorders in children with autism and mental retardation and in blind people; and possibly effective in case of jet-lag, sunburns and preoperative anxiety.

"However, other studies which use melatonin as medication show its high level of effectiveness," Darío Acuña-Castroviejo explains to SINC. He has been studying melatonin for several years at the Health Sciences Technology Park of the University of Granada.

The expert points out that international consensus already exists, promoted by the British Association for Psychopharmacology--also published in the *Journal of Psychopharmacology* in 2010–which has melatonin as the first choice treatment for insomnia in patients above the age of 55. This consensus is now being transferred to cases of insomnia in children.

Its use in treating neurodegenerative diseases is acquiring increasing scientific support in lateral amyotrophic sclerosis, in Alzheimer's, and Duchenne muscular dystrophy.

"Even though many more studies and clinical tests are still required to assess the doses of melatonin which will be effective for a wide range of diseases, the antioxidant and anti-inflammatory properties of melatonin mean that its use is highly recommended for diseases which feature oxidative stress and inflammation," Acuña-Castroviejo states.

This is the case for diseases such as epilepsy, chronic fatigue, fibromyalgia, and even the aging process itself, where data is available pointing to the benefits of melatonin, though said data is not definitive.

Reference:

García-Mesa Y, Giménez-Llort L, López LC, Venegas C, Cristòfol R, Escames G, Acuña-Castroviejo D, Sanfeliu C. "Melatonin plus physical exercise are highly neuroprotective in the 3xTg-AD mouse". *Neurobiol Aging* 2012 Jun; 33(6):1124.e13-29.

One more exciting thing:
My lab results for my blood test after I had been taking
about 300 mg a night of melatonin for around two months
showed that my LH levels dropped by 30% (from 6.9 to 4.9
[mIU/mL]) and my FSH levels by 13% (from 8.8 to
7.7[mIU/mL]). So the prediction seems to be true--
melatonin really suppresses LH. I am a little disappointed
that the FSH did not drop further. Maybe I will need to
explore the idea of trying follistatin which selectively
suppresses FSH.

I did another test to see if the melatonin boosted my
progesterone levels. My progesterone rose from 1.9 to 2.2
ng/ml by taking melatonin, a nice 15% increase. However,
my starting pre-melatonin progesterone level of 1.9 was
already way higher than the upper limit of the reference
range of 1.4 for men. (I believe this is due to my habit of
taking 100 mg of pregnenolone a day, which is a direct
precursor to progesterone.) So my progesterone levels are
sky-high while taking pregnenolone, and go even higher
while taking melatonin! As predicted--thank you very
much.

As you already know, men and women are very different
from a sexual/physical point of view. This goes the same
for their hormones, even though the sex hormones are the
same in both males and females. (For example both men

and women make estrogen and testosterone, but their levels are extremely different.) The sex hormone levels between the sexes vary dramatically! For example, women in their 20's to 40's have about 10 times the LH levels that men have, and $1/10^{th}$ the testosterone--and way more estrogen!

If LH attacks the brain and causes Alzheimer's, how can women survive such high levels (compared to men) of LH their whole lives? My best guess, and the best guess of a researcher at the University of Wisconsin and former employee/major stockholder of Voyager Pharmaceuticals, Craig Atwood (who was not involved in Dr. Bowen's original patent application for suppressing LH to treat AD), is that women's very high levels of progesterone protect their brain from the effects of high LH. But after age 40, when their LH levels shoot sky-high by 1,000s of percent, then the progesterone can no longer protect the brain from the LH attack. (An interesting fact to consider that somewhat supports the idea of LH attacking the brain is that many more women than men live to age 90 and older. However, the men that make it to age 90 and beyond are rarely demented, while women who become this old are overwhelmingly demented. Could it be due to a lifetime of much higher LH levels in women than men?)

My theory suggests that while LH attacks the brain, progesterone *protects* the brain. But in men, there apparently is not much of an LH attack. Thus, suppressing LH does not alter the course of AD very much in men.

One thing I noticed in my research about hormones and aging, was that in men, the hormones estradiol, progesterone, LH, and FSH all seem to go up a little bit every decade on average. But all of a sudden, at around age 70, progesterone levels start to decline in the average man, whereas they had been on a lifelong rise up to that time.

When this happens, LH and FSH levels just start to skyrocket, increasing way faster than before. Thus, I got the idea that a drop in progesterone in men was a hormonal signal to kill them off by suppressing the protective effects of progesterone, AND increasing the two "bad" hormones LH and FSH.

I looked into progesterone a little more, and found that one of the most fascinating facts about it is that it is one of the best neuroprotective substances on earth. There are tons of studies that show women survive traumatic brain injuries much better than men because of their high progesterone levels.

So, this is the theory that I finally came up with and had detailed in my 3rd published paper--which ultimately explained the odd results of the Voyager experiment where

Lupron only stopped AD in women, and not men!

LH attacks the brain--Progesterone protects the brain

High levels of LH in women cause AD by an increased attack on the brain. Low levels of progesterone in men cause AD by a decreased protection/repair of the brain.

So that's it. You now have all the treatments known to man that actually stop Alzheimer's in its tracks. Treatments such as Lupron and melatonin have some evidence suggesting their effectiveness, while using progesterone in men still remains a theory--but a very good one, which awaits confirmation by some of you readers giving it a try and reporting back. Please contact me at JEFFBO AT AOL DOT COM (I spelled out the "at" and the "dot" so the computer robots will not trash me with spam) and let me know your plans and any results you get, and I will add you to my database.

Chapter Four—Pharmaceuticals for Alzheimer's?

The main prescription drugs you can get from Big Pharma for Alzheimer's are pathetic and do very little, from what I know. One class is *acetylcholinestrase inhibitors*. How do these drugs work? All brains have acetylcholine, a neurotransmitter. But they also have chemicals called acetylcholinesterases. When they add "ase" to a chemical term, it means it is an enzyme--a chemical that activates a chemical reaction. So an acetylcholinester-ase just chops up acetylcholine. And an inhibitor of this molecule prevents the "ase" from chopping up acetylcholine. The current theory is that because acetylcholine levels go down in Alzheimer's patients' brains, if acetylcholine levels rose by preventing its destruction, it should help AD patients.

From Wikipedia:

Most indirect-acting ACh receptor agonists work by inhibiting the enzyme acetylcholinesterase. The resulting accumulation of acetylcholine causes continuous stimulation of the muscles, glands, and central nervous system.

They are examples of *enzyme inhibitors*, and increase the action of acetylcholine by delaying its degradation; some have been used as *nerve agents (Sarin* and *VX nerve gas)* or pesticides (organophosphates and the carbamates). In clinical use, they are administered to reverse the action of muscle relaxants, to treat myasthenia gravis, and to treat symptoms of Alzheimer's disease (rivastigmine, which increases cholinergic activity in the brain).

The bottom line is, one of Big Pharma's treatments for AD is basically giving patients a variant of *nerve gas*! As you might expect, it doesn't work all that well.

From: Alzheimer's Disease--Causes, Stages, and Symptoms, by Howard Crystal MD

Another theory they have is that glutamate is the major excitatory neurotransmitter in the brain. One theory suggests that too much glutamate may be bad for the brain and cause deterioration of nerve cells. Memantine (*Namenda*) works by partially decreasing the effect of glutamate to activate nerve cells. It has not been proven that memantine slows down the rate of progression of Alzheimer's disease. Studies have demonstrated that some patients on memantine can care for themselves better than patients on sugar pills (placebos). Memantine is approved for treatment of moderate and severe dementia, and studies did not show it was helpful in mild dementia.

Existing Drugs for Alzheimer's

Aricept

What It Is: One of the most widely used drugs to treat the symptoms of disease. Aricept is FDA-approved for mild, moderate, and severe stages of the disease.

How It Works: Aricept is a cholinesterase inhibitor that prevents the breakdown of acetylcholine in the brain. Acetylcholine plays a key role in memory and learning; higher levels in the brain help nerve cells communicate more efficiently.

Effectiveness: Aricept postpones the worsening of Alzheimer's symptoms for 6 to 12 months in about half of the people who take it. For many, the improvement is minimal, yet worthwhile. Anecdotal evidence suggests that a small percentage of people may benefit more dramatically from this drug.

Dosage: Aricept is available in tablet form or an orally disintegrating tablet form, and is commonly started at 5 mg a day. If it's well tolerated after 4 to 6 weeks, the dosage may be increased to 10 mg a day. Your health care professional will determine the best dosage for you or your loved one.

Side Effects: Although generally well-tolerated, the most common side effects are nausea, diarrhea, increased frequency of bowel movements, vomiting, bruising, sleep disturbance, muscle cramps, loss of appetite, fatigue, and fainting.

Exelon

What It Is: A commonly used drug to treat the symptoms of Alzheimer's disease Exelon is FDA approved for mild and moderate stages of the disease; it is also approved for the treatment of mild to moderate dementia due to Parkinson's disease.

How It Works: Exelon is a cholinesterase inhibitor that prevents the breakdown of acetylcholine and butyrylcholine in the brain by blocking the activity of two different enzymes. Acetylcholine and butyrylcholine play a key role in memory and learning; higher levels in the brain help nerve cells communicate more efficiently.

Effectiveness: Exelon postpones the worsening of Alzheimer's symptoms for 6 to 12 months in about half of the people who take it. For many, the improvement is minimal, yet worthwhile. Anecdotal evidence suggests that a small percentage of people may benefit more dramatically from this drug.

Dosage: Exelon is available as a capsule, liquid, and patch. In capsule or liquid form, it's commonly started at 1.5 mg twice a day; if it's well-tolerated, the capsule or liquid dosage is increased by 3 mg a day every two weeks until the dosage reaches 6 mg twice a day. In patch form, a 4.6 mg, 5 cm patch is worn once a day for 4 weeks. If it's well-tolerated, the dosage may be increased to a 9.5 mg, 10 cm patch once a day. Your healthcare professional will determine the best dosage for you or your loved one.

Side Effects: The most common side effects of Exelon are nausea, diarrhea, increased frequency of bowel movements, vomiting, muscle weakness, loss of appetite, weight loss, dizziness, drowsiness, and upset stomach. People who weigh less than 110 pounds may experience more severe side effects and may need to stop taking Exelon.

Razadyne (galantamine HBr)

What It Is: A drug used to treat the symptoms of Alzheimer's disease. Razadyne (galantamine HBr) is FDA-approved for mild and moderate stages of the disease.

How It Works: In technical terms, Razadyne is a cholinesterase inhibitor that prevents the breakdown of acetylcholine in the brain. Acetylcholine plays a key role in memory and learning; higher levels in the brain help nerve cells communicate more efficiently. Razadyne also stimulates nicotinic receptors to release more acetylcholine in the brain.

Effectiveness: Razadyne delays the worsening of Alzheimer's symptoms for 6 to 12 months in about half of the people who take it. For many, the improvement is minimal, yet worthwhile. Anecdotal evidence suggests that a small percentage of people may benefit more dramatically from this drug.

Dosage: Razadyne is available in tablet and capsule form, and is commonly started at 4 mg twice a day. If it's well tolerated after 4 weeks, the dosage may be increased to 8 mg twice a day. After another four weeks, the dosage may be increased to 12 mg twice a day. Razadyne also comes in an extended release, once-a-day tablet (Razadyne ER). Your health care professional will determine the best dosage for you or your loved one.

Namenda

What It Is: One of the newer drugs used to treat the symptoms of Alzheimer's disease. Namenda is FDA-approved for moderate and severe stages of the disease.

How It Works: In technical terms, Namenda is an N-methyl D-aspartate (NMDA) antagonist that regulates the activity of glutamate in the brain. Glutamate plays a key role in memory and learning, but excess glutamate can lead to the disruption of nerve cell communication or nerve cell death.

Effectiveness: Studies involving Namenda have shown that the drug can slow the rate of decline in thinking and the ability to perform daily activities in individuals who have moderate to severe Alzheimer's disease. For many, the improvement is minimal, yet worthwhile.

Dosage: Namenda is available in tablet and liquid form and is commonly started at 5 mg a day. If it's well tolerated, the dosage may be gradually increased -- at a minimum of one-week intervals -- to 5 mg twice a day, 15 mg/day (5 mg and 10 mg separately), and 10 mg twice a day. Your health care professional will determine the best dosage for you or your loved one.

Side Effects: Although generally well-tolerated, the most common side effects are dizziness, headache, constipation, and confusion. Unlike cholinesterase inhibitors such as Aricept, Exelon, and Razadyne, those taking Namenda have a low risk of gastrointestinal side effects.

Medications for early to moderate stages

All of the prescription medications currently approved to treat Alzheimer's symptoms in early to moderate stages are from a class of drugs called cholinesterase inhibitors. Cholinesterase inhibitors are prescribed to treat symptoms related to memory, thinking, language, judgment and other thought processes. Prevent the breakdown of acetylcholine (a-SEA-til-KOH-lean), a chemical messenger important for learning and memory. This supports communication among nerve cells by keeping acetylcholine levels high.

- Delay worsening of symptoms for 6 to 12 months, on average, for about half the people who take them.
- Are generally well tolerated. If side effects occur, they commonly include nausea, vomiting, loss of appetite and increased frequency of bowel movements.

Three cholinesterase inhibitors are commonly prescribed:

- Donepezil (Aricept) is approved to treat all stages of Alzheimer's.
- Rivastigmine (Exelon) is approved to treat mild to moderate Alzheimer's.
- Galantamine (Razadyne) is approved to treat mild to moderate Alzheimer's.

Tacrine (Cognex) was the first cholinesterase inhibitor approved. Doctors rarely prescribe it today because it's associated with more serious side effects than the other three drugs in this class.

Medication for moderate to severe stages

A second type of medication, memantine (Namenda) is approved by the FDA for treatment of moderate to severe Alzheimer's.

Memantine is prescribed to improve memory, attention, reason, language and the ability to perform simple tasks. It can be used alone or with other Alzheimer's disease treatments. There is some evidence that individuals with moderate to severe Alzheimer's who are taking a cholinesterase inhibitor might benefit by also taking memantine. Donepezil (Aricept) is the only cholinesterase inhibitor approved to treat all stages of Alzheimer's disease, including moderate to severe.

Memantine:

- Regulates the activity of glutamate, a different messenger chemical involved in learning and memory.

- Delays worsening of symptoms for some people temporarily. Many experts consider its benefits similar to those of cholinesterase inhibitors.
- Can cause side effects, including headache, constipation, confusion and dizziness.

That's about *all* Big Pharma has for us for AD--two types of drugs, where *none* of them have been shown to work much at all.

Chapter Five—*More* Treatment Regimens for Alzheimer's that *Work*

The two treatments I've described for AD patients--suppressing LH via Lupron and melatonin both seem to work in very small studies (if you want to call the twins observation a study), and both are based on the latest cutting edge theory on AD which is now being championed by scientists at the NIH. These two treatments also jibe well with the idea that purposeful hormones drive the aging process, not random evolutionary mistakes.

These two treatments, Lupron and melatonin, I believe give you way better odds for a successful outcome than you are going to get from your orthodox physician or from Big Pharma. These two treatments have been shown to be effective on a very small scale in both men and women (and now in mice-for melatonin). Neither of these treatments are of interest to Big Pharma because they would never generate profits. Best of all, to get melatonin you don't even need a doctor's prescription--you just get it over the counter or off the internet. If you are going to take high doses of melatonin, it is best to find a bulk supplier of the hormone like Vitaspace at www.Vitaspace.com, which sells melatonin in bulk. You can get 1 kilogram for $300, or 30 cents a gram. That's a lot better than buying the 3 mg pills which can cost you $40 a gram! Lupron might be a bit trickier, but any doctor can order it for you off-the-shelf, and if you are diligent enough, you can probably find it on the internet without a need for a prescription.

A third treatment that I recommend is still theoretical, and it is up to us to give it a try--*progesterone for men*. Big Pharma will never test progesterone since they can't make much money off it--nor will they test melatonin, for the same reason. Lupron injections also will have little appeal to Big Pharma--look what a mess Voyager made of this promising treatment.

One additional hormone that you can get over the counter that I expect would be just as effective as progesterone is a hormone called *pregnenolone* (see Appendix I). Pregnenolone is the precursor to progesterone and a host of other steroidal hormones, including DHEA, testosterone and estradiol, amongst others. Pregnenolone is also known as the "memory" hormone, and is the one hormone that when given to rats has a dramatic positive effect on their memories. Pregnenolone has been shown to boost the memory of very old rats to equal the memory of the youngest, healthiest rats. Another reported effect of pregnenolone is that it causes those who take it to overcome social shyness. Finally, pregnenolone stimulates the production of *acetylcholine*. You know, the neurotransmitter that most of the Alzheimer's drugs are trying to boost--by preventing the breakdown of acetylcholine by inhibiting acetylcholinesterase (basically a scissor-like enzyme that snips acetylcholine into pieces).

Why don't the drug companies also treat Alzheimer's by boosting acetylcholine production with pregnenolone? Take a wild guess--they can't patent it, so there is no money in it. You can get pregnenolone cheaply from the Life Extension Foundation, which I encourage everyone to join who is interested in their health. They are cutting- edge and are about 20 years ahead of almost any doctor you will encounter. When you join, you get their excellent monthly magazine which has given me many important clues for my theories. Their website address is www.lef.org.

The bottom line is, if I was a woman in the initial stages of AD I would run to the store to get melatonin and start taking a minimum of 75 mg a night, and might even boost it up to 500 mg a night! There has *never* been any toxicity associated with it yet, although I know of some side effects about which I will tell you later.

The same advice goes for men just starting out with AD-- except boost the dose of melatonin to 125 mg minimum (since men usually weigh more), and go higher if you want.

I would also start taking 200 to 400 mg a day of pregnenolone, and the same amount of progesterone. You can get 100 mg pregnenolone pills from www.lef.org pretty cheaply. I have never bought progesterone pills (*Prometrium*, 100 and 200 mg).

In either case, with high dose melatonin, get prepared to sleep (like I did) 14 hours a day for 4 months or so--but the sleep feels really good. Then, if you are like me, you will get back to sleeping 7 hours a day while still maintaining a high dose of melatonin. I know about this because about 10 years ago I performed the same experiment on myself, taking up to 500 mg of melatonin every night for a year. One nice side effect: it made my thinning hair grow back thick.

It would be best to boost your melatonin doses gradually--get used to 3 mg, over a week or so, then go to 6 mg, for a week, then 12 mg, etc etc, doubling the dose every time you get used to the old dose. Why?

I've had friends go right to 100 mg or so, and they would get no effect for the first night nor the second day. Then, all of a sudden, on the third day they would get so dizzy they could not easily walk, and freaked out. A similar thing happened to a friend of mine who had really high blood pressure, something like 200/140. I put him on high-dose melatonin right off the bat. Day 1, nothing happened. Day 2, his blood pressure dropped by 50 points on both scales, but he said when he was on the bus he got really dizzy and really sleepy. So unfortunately, he got scared off, quit taking melatonin, went back on his doctor's drugs, and eventually had a stroke from his high blood pressure and died. This was not unexpected, since he had been suffering from kidney failure and was on dialysis. High blood pressure and death by stroke is common for these kidney patients.

The bottom line protocol I suggest you try to stop Alzheimer's in both men and women is as follows:

Gradually boost the dose of melatonin from 3 mg a night for the first week to 6 mg for the second, then 12 mg the third week, then 24 mg the fourth, 48 mg the fifth, to 75 mg a night for women in the sixth. For men, boost melatonin to 96 mg in the fifth week, and then 120 mg the 7th week. Women--stay on 75 mg for the rest of your life; men--stay on 120 mg for the rest of your life. If you want, you can boost it up to 500 mg a night without many worries, as it is totally nontoxic, but might have some side effects.

From the first week, also take at least 2 doses of 100mg of DHEA day and night, 2 doses of 100 mg of pregnenolone, day and night, and 2 does of 100 mg of progesterone, day and night.

If you continue to see a decline on your loved one with AD, you could also add high-dose Lupron injections, but I would do this as a last resort, due to the side effects and cost.

I believe this will be your best bet to combat this once hopeless and horrifying disease (and now treatable, we hope). What Big Pharma and your doctors have for you just will not work and is not based on the latest cutting edge theory.

Please email me with your results at jeffbo AT aol DOT com. I changed the @ to AT and the "." to DOT so that computer robots will not grab my email address and inundate me with spam!

Here are two emails I received from a reader who is trying the protocol with her husband who was recently diagnosed with AD:
November 7th:

" I downloaded your book on my Kindle app on my ipad. My husband, who is 78, was diagnosed early AD in September of this year. The doctor prescribed Aricept, and the pharmacy filled it with Donepizil, 10 mg at night. The doctor said to split the 10 mg in half for the first week, and if there were no side effects, to start taking the whole pill. His intellect is still good. He still reads the Wall Street Journal. It's his short term memory that was the problem. He did seem a little better on the new medication, but still repeated things over and over.

I gave him a 3 mg Melatonin Monday night. Yesterday, he did not repeat anything. Nor has he today. He seems more with it. You most probably are rolling your eyes. His sense of humor is better.

There has been no side effect, so I intend to increase his Melatonin to two 3mg pills tomorrow night.

He had prostate cancer 17 years ago, and received the seed radiation treatment. His PSA tests have been like .001 for the past 10 years. I hesitate to give him Pregnenolone, because of his prostate cancer history. He is going to his urologist in the next week or so and we'll ask him.

Thank you for your book. I hope this continues to work. "

December 8th-

"He's up to 20 mg of melatonin a night plus 50 mg of pregnenolone, plus his 10 mg of Donepezil (Aricept generic). His memory has not gotten worse, and I see an improvement in his sense of humor, which used to be wonderful. But had gotten a little dull. He seems to want to tease me more which he had completely stopped. He still continues to drive beautifully. He does ask me to help him with locations of places we are going, but once I jog his memory, he says, Oh yes--I remember. He still has moments of short term memory loss, but they aren't as plentiful....or they don't seem so to me.

I think he is showing some improvement. When can I join your group?"

I will post updates of this case as the info comes in:

The Group in question above is a Yahoo group: http://health.groups.yahoo.com/group/AlzheimersCanBeStoppedNow/
Please join this group if you have any interest in experiments with melatonin and pregnenolone for Alzheimer's. Everyone's participation is needed. Thank you!

I was motivated to write this book by two of my friends emailing me and asking me how best to treat Alzheimer's-one of them had recently heard of the coconut oil cure. I know nothing about the coconut oil cure, so I add it here. Why? Because unlike most scientists, I am willing to say "maybe" instead of "no." Maybe it works? And I would expect it is not dangerous--thus give it a try and add it to the melatonin and other things. I am skeptical however, because if Alzheimer's is a disease caused by your hormones, which evidence is mounting that this is true--

then I would expect the best cure for Alzheimer's to be found in other hormones that combat the "bad" hormones.

Caprylic acid (clinically tested as Ketasyn [AC-1202], marketed as a "medical food" called Axona®) and coconut oil

Caprylic acid is the active ingredient of Axona, which is marketed as a "medical food." Caprylic acid is a medium-chain triglyceride (fat) produced by processing coconut oil or palm kernel oil. The body breaks down caprylic acid into substances called "ketone bodies." The theory behind Axona is that the ketone bodies derived from caprylic acid may provide an alternative energy source for brain cells that have lost their ability to use glucose (sugar) as a result of Alzheimer's. Glucose is the brain's chief energy source. Imaging studies show reduced glucose use in brain regions affected by Alzheimer's.

Axona's development was preceded by development of the chemically similar Ketasyn (AC-1202). Ketasyn was tested in a Phase II clinical study enrolling 152 volunteers with mild to moderate Alzheimer's. Most participants were also taking FDA-approved Alzheimer's drugs The manufacturer of Axona reports that study participants who took Ketasyn performed better on tests of memory and overall function than those who received a placebo (a look-alike, inactive treatment).

The chief goal of Phase II studies is about the safety and best dose of an experimental treatment. Phase II trials are generally too small to confirm that a treatment works. To demonstrate effectiveness under the prescription drug approval framework, the FDA requires drug developers to follow Phase II studies with larger Phase III trials enrolling several hundred to thousands of volunteers.

The manufacturer of Ketasyn decided not to conduct Phase III studies to confirm its effectiveness. The company chose instead to use Ketasyn as the basis of Axona and promote Axona as a "medical food." Medical foods do not require Phase III studies or any other clinical testing. The Alzheimer's Association Medical and Scientific Advisory Council has expressed concern that there is not enough evidence to assess the potential benefit of medical foods for Alzheimer's disease. For more information, please see the Medical and Scientific Advisory Council statement about medical foods.

Some people with Alzheimer's and their caregivers have turned to coconut oil as a less expensive, over-the-counter source of caprylic acid. A few people have reported that coconut oil helped the person with Alzheimer's, but there's never been any clinical testing of coconut oil for Alzheimer's, and there's no scientific evidence that it helps.

I will update this book periodically, so it is best for you to get the most recent copy, where I will tell you all of results that are reported to me.

Here is an INTERESTNG UPDATE! I could not shake the feeling that somehow eating coconut oil actually helps Alzheimer's patients by altering their hormones in some way. A friend of mine who had never taken supplements before decided to try a little experiment. He tested his blood for the hormones pregnenolone, progesterone, and Vitamin D3 before he started **eating 3 tablespoons of coconut oil a day for a month.** After a month of coconut oil he went back and tested the hormones again. I was surprised that his progesterone did not increase, and was not surprised that his Vitamin D3 levels remain unchanged. **I was absolutely ecstatic when the test revealed that his pregnenolone levels had increased by 250%!** So maybe there is something to the coconut oil Alzheimer's hypothesis after all! And if it works it is likely working by a completely different manner than most researchers suggest. I am now much more optimistic about the efficacy of coconut oil for Alzheimer's than before. Admittedly, I was a bit disappointed that his progesterone levels did not change. However, my friend that did this experiment was 32 years old at the time and his progesterone levels in the beginning of the study were already towards the highest level of the reference range for men. I am hoping that in older people with much lower progesterone levels that eating coconut oil might boost not only their pregnenolone levels but progesterone levels as well. Future testing will resolve this question. If you want to do the test yourself you can get blood tests cheaply and easily at www.lef.org. If you do the test please report back to me-thanks.

Chapter Six--Melatonin

I discovered the possible source of the dizziness when I used to fast for 3 days at a time, eating no calories at all. If I had not been fasting for a while, I was usually dizzy when I woke up on the morning of the third day. It was the same dizziness I experienced when I had not been taking melatonin for a long time, and went right into the high doses. Thus, I believe, the dizziness some people get from going to high-dose melatonin right off the bat is the same dizziness you get from starvation. The dizziness took 3 days to kick in with me when I was fasting, but I got it in one day when going to high-dose melatonin out of the blue.

What is melatonin? There are a lot of books out there that you can read, but I will give you a brief synopsis.

Melatonin is a hormone that most living creatures make. It is basically the CLOCK hormone that controls the production of all your other hormones. It is a super-strong antioxidant and an interesting little chemical. Its structure looks like it is almost trying to imitate many of the steroid hormones like testosterone, DHEA, estradiol, estrone, progesterone, pregnenolone, cortisol, or Vitamin D3.

Here is melatonin's structure: Here is the steroid DHEA:

And just for fun here is Vitamin D3's structure:

vitamin D

Below, we show cholesterol and how it is transformed into all the steroidal hormones. It looks like melatonin is trying to be a steroid--but just not quite making it.

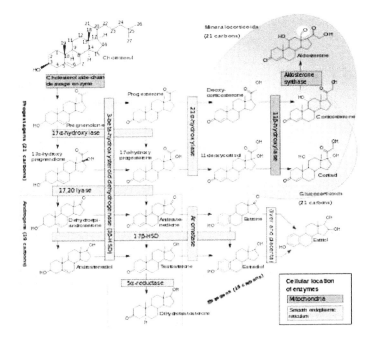

Steroidogenesis with enzymes and intermediates

Melatonin is produced by the pineal gland at night. It is called the *pineal gland* because it looks like a little pine cone, where it sits just under your brain.

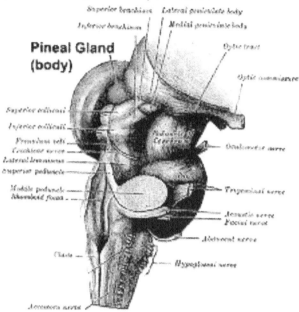

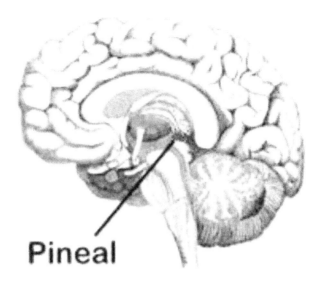

Pineal

I've found that melatonin drives the increase of most of your "good" hormones, and suppresses most of your "bad" hormones. Melatonin also suppresses your reproductive hormones regardless of whether they are bad or good. That's why it can be used for birth control.

Babies have really high levels of melatonin. That is why babies sleep so much. If you take a lot of melatonin for awhile, you will also find that your skin gets as soft as a baby's and your ears get really flexible--also like a baby's. Melatonin suppresses most sex- related hormones like FSH,

LH, testosterone and estrogen. And it suppresses your sex drive! It also makes injuries and bruises take a lot longer to heal. I think it slows down the rate at which your cells divide, and in this way might slow the aging process. Adding melatonin to the drinking water of mice increases their average lifespan by 20%. High levels of melatonin are what keep young children from going into puberty. As the melatonin levels drop with age, the gonadotropic hormones LH and FSH increase and drive the process of puberty. (Thus, one use for Lupron is to suppress accelerated (precocious) puberty, since it also suppresses LH and FSH, just like melatonin!). Melatonin peaks at night, and the peaks keep dropping throughout your life, and can drop to 60% by the time you hit age 50!!

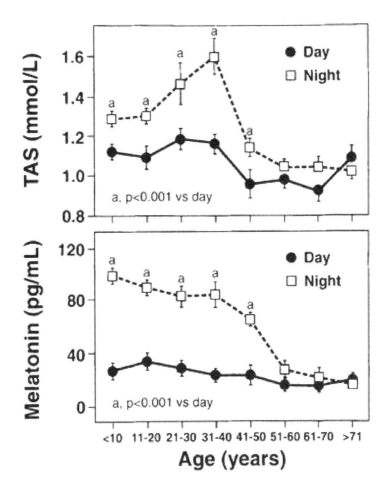

Figure 4.
Age-related changes in day and night melatonin levels and the total antioxidant status (TAS) of the blood of humans at

various ages. In this study, the individuals, ranging in age from 2 to 89 years, were categorized into 10-year bins. As described previously, increased age is associated with a reduction in nocturnal melatonin values; this drop correlates with a reduction in the TAS of the blood. This suggests that as melatonin is lost, the ability of individuals to resist oxidative damage is likewise lessened. From Benot *et al.*

Around age 50, levels of LH and FSH start to increase out of control, and I believe attack your body to kill you. One reason this likely happens is because of the drop in melatonin that occurs with age. Why? Melatonin suppresses the production of LH and FSH.

Side Effects of High-Dose Melatonin

You have heard about my year-long experience with high-dose melatonin. Other things that I should add about my experiment is that it made me dream a lot. And it also dramatically reduced my sex drive and sex production. And it made my thinning hair grow back nice and thick.

Now I do have to warn you of some unpleasant side effects that a few of my friends trying high dose melatonin have experienced.

In women who have bald fathers, high-dose melatonin

really made their hair start to thin and fall out--Not to the point of balding, but they lost about half their hair thickness, and usually stopped due to the effect. If women had fathers with full heads of hair, high-dose melatonin did not affect their hair. However, if you are a woman with beginning Alzheimer's, I would think losing your hair versus losing your mind would be a choice that you would make. You can always get a nice wig.

I have also noticed that if one has the shingles virus hiding in one's DNA, melatonin can trigger it into coming out. Shingles is kind of nasty. It creates a circle of little bumps like a flower that develop on the skin, on one side of the body. These little bumps become like weepy little pimples that hurt and ooze a fluid. They occur in people who have had chicken pox, which lasts a lifetime. Two people I know of who took high-dose melatonin got shingles. Both quit when they broke out with shingles. I do not know if you can keep taking it and get through the shingles, or not. But if you had to choose Alzheimer's vs. shingles, I would guess you would choose shingles.

I also know of a woman who took high-dose melatonin who suddenly got a months-long problem that seemed like Lyme disease that might have also been hiding in her DNA. So for some people, high-dose melatonin will be a blessing, and in some it will be both a blessing and a curse. It depends on what's hiding in your DNA. But if one wants to avoid the progression of Alzheimer's, I would expect that these problems will seem somewhat minor. In my small experience, it seems about 20% of the people will have some of these undesired side effects caused by triggering hidden viruses in their DNA. But if it stops Alzheimer's in its tracks, I expect one will have to just go with it.

Chapter Seven—Origins of Aging: Evolution, Cells, Plants, and Animals—Influence of Hormones

Just like a plant that has flowered and dropped its seeds starts to rapidly decay due to changes in its hormones, the melatonin decline really accelerates right before, during, and after the age of menopause in females (from 50 to 60).

In a way, we are similar to annual plants. After we have reproduced and no longer can have any more kids (as a female), our hormones turn on us to destroy us. You can test this idea (in plants, at least) by growing some annual plants (a plant that only lives one year) and letting some develop flowers and seeds while snipping off any of the reproductive organs developing on other plants. Then just watch and see how the two groups of plants react over time. You will see the non-reproducing plants go on living happy and growing while the plants that have reproduced "go to seed" and self-destruct via action of various hormones. In fact, it used to be a law in the United States that all tobacco growers were required to remove the flowers and stamens from all tobacco plants grown for smoking tobacco to make sure the US had the best tobacco leaf in the world!

I believe humans, as well as almost all other animals, display a slow-motion variation of this life cycle theme that is so obvious in annual plants. (Of course, men can still reproduce long after age 50, but that is just a little complication to the big picture I present which applies to most mammals, whose males usually die at about the same time females lose their reproductive capacity. Humans are an odd exception, where the female goes on living long after menopause, and the male lifespan matches her long lifespan.)

My theory is that the human female has evolved such a long post-reproductive life (as high as 70 years after her first 50 years, if she lives to 120) so that her sons could enjoy a longer reproductive life (assuming they inherit her aging system). Thus, from this line of reasoning, humans started off with the typical mammalian life history where both the male and female generally do not live much longer than the point where the female undergoes reproductive senescence (menopause)--around age 50. In humans, longer lifespan after menopause has been selected for and has led to this strange situation. How was life after menopause selected for? The human invention of kings seems to have caused the evolution of long life spans that continue long after the end of the female's reproductive life of 50 years. If the mother of a king evolved a longer post-menopausal lifespan and gave that longer lifespan to her son, her son could then go on fathering many more children than if he died off at age 50. (A huge evolutionary advantage if the goal of evolution is generally to maximize the spread of genes.) If you doubt me on this, just check how many people in Asia carry genes from Genghis Kahn. Or look up how many children the famous Pharaoh Ramses sired in his 90 some-odd years. I call it the son-king hypothesis, a nice play on the sun-king idea of ancient religions.

It might also be interesting to speculate about why women endure a crash in their progesterone levels at the age of menopause (50-ish) while the progesterone levels of men tend to keep increasing each year until they reach an age of about 70 and that is when the male progesterone crash begins. One might expect that before post reproductive lifespans evolved for females and thus were inherited by males, that both sexes experienced the progesterone crash at about the same age (50). This rise in male progesterone from age 50 to age 70 might just be the thing that evolved to allow him a reproductive life after the age of 50. Additionally if progesterone protects the brain, this might also explain why women who live to age 90 are usually demented while any man reaching this age is generally sharp as a tack.

Now our eminent scientists, stuck in their logical boxes, can only come up with the "grandmother hypothesis" to explain why human females live so long after their reproductive life ends. Their thinking is that somehow grandma helps her daughters raise the daughters' children better and increases their odds of survival, so therefore "MENOPAUSE IS DIRECTLY SELECTED FOR."

They can find no statistical evidence that this is true, and if you ask me, it is a ridiculous stretch and defies all forms of common sense. There is an implicit assumption in this idea that women used to live to 120 and were able to reproduce during the entire 120 years. And then menopause came along, got them to quit having children at age 50, so they could help their daughters' children survive better for the next 70 years. Preposterous!

If menopause is selected for, it cannot be at the individual level, but *must* be at the group level, and is actually the evolutionary remnant of what most mammals and other animals endure--rapid aging and death that occur with reproductive decline. (It seems evolution doesn't want individuals to reproduce too much, which would reduce the species diversity. Thus, we can see how aging and reproductive decline would be linked.) Mainstream scientists/theorists cannot accept group selection as an evolutionary force due to their being stuck in their logical box. More on this later.

It all seems so complicated in us "higher" organisms. Let's take a look at the simplest forms of life to see if things are more clear. There is a kingdom of life called bacteria, or *prokaryotes*, that in general are single-cell organisms. These organisms have DNA, but instead of chromosomes (which are linear) have plasmids, or *circles* of DNA, with no beginning and no end, that just float around in the single cell.

Now mammals, other animals and plants, belong to a different group of life called the *eukaryotes*, which keep DNA locked away inside a cell nucleus which resides inside the single cell. There are many forms of eukaryote single cell life. Remember, *all* eukaryotes, whether single-cell organisms or more complicated multi-cell organisms all have one thing in common--**linear** DNA, also known as *chromosomes* (as opposed to circular bacterial plasmid DNA). One interesting thing about linear DNA is that it is bad for the organism because when DNA is copied, it cannot be copied all the way to the end of the chromosome--there is not enough room. It is called the "end replication problem." So chromosomes shrink every time the cell divides, and when they shrink enough, DNA with essential genes is not copied and the cell dies (or so the theory goes –it is likely more complicated and much more controlled than this).

So we can see that the most simple single cell eukaryotic organisms start off with an aging system (chromosome-shortening) that is triggered by reproduction (cell division) (since DNA has to be copied, and thus the chromosomes shorten every time the cell divides, is the same as saying the cell reproduces). In this case, it is so obvious that aging and reproduction are two sides of the same coin, and that reproduction drives aging. All, I am doing is taking this simple concept and showing how it is also true in the obvious examples of aging/reproduction in annual plants, Pacific Salmon, bamboo, etc., and then suggesting that it might also be going on in more complicated animals.

If you remain unconvinced that sex-related hormones can cause aging and death after your annual plant experiment, then just read up on what are called the "semalparous" reproducing species to gain a little more insight. The Pacific Salmon, the female octopus, marsupial mice--there are actually a reasonable number of these examples, but mainstream evolutionary theorists like to put these obvious cases of programmed hormonal aging into a special category where they can then be ignored!!!

If you read comments from the "experts" in the field of aging, you will often see them actually saying these instances of programmed/reproductive aging do not represent real aging. I heard this direct from Aubrey de Grey, a popular aging guru. Anyway, let's not get too far into the origin of the aging debate. That is plenty enough material for another book.

Here are some more detailed examples of how various organisms are caused to age and die by the action of their reproductive hormones, so it will be easier for you to envision how the same processes of increases in reproduction-related hormones might be going on within us to age us, give us aging related diseases, and eventually cause us to wither and die.

Aging in Annual Plants:

There are two main types of plants that gardeners classify--the annuals and the perennials. Annual plants sprout grow, blossom, and die all in one year. While the perennials might lose leaves and go dormant in the winter, but they come back to life the next season. Let us just look at annuals for now to keep things simple.

From Wikipedia:

Plant senescence is the study of aging in plants. It is a heavily studied subject just as it is in the other kingdoms of life. Plants, just like other forms of organisms, seem to have both unintended and programmed aging. Leaf senescence is the cause of autumn leaf color in deciduous trees.

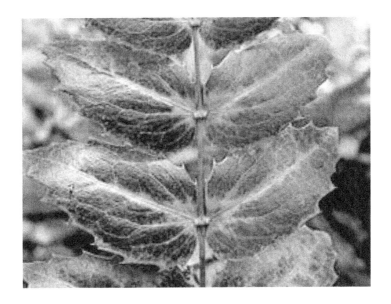

The autumn senescence of Oregon Grape leaves is an example of *programmed* plant senescence.

Programmed senescence

Programmed senescence seems to be heavily influenced by plant hormones. The hormones abscisic acid and ethylene are accepted by most scientists as the main causes, but at least one source believes gibberellins and brassinosteroids are equally responsible. Cytokinins help to maintain the plant cell but when they are withdrawn or if the cell can not receive the cytokinin it may then undergo apoptosis or senescence.

Since I don't know all that much about plant aging and plant hormones, I leave this as a test for you to probe the assumptions in my theory. I will bet that all the hormones in plants involved with aging are also involved with development and reproduction. Let me know what you find out. I am so confident that reproductive hormones also become pro-aging hormones that I will throw this out there without actually knowing the correct answer--but being willing to bet my reputation that you will find my guess correct! Go for it. Make my day!

Aging in the Perennial Bamboo Plant (from Wikipedia)

Mass flowering

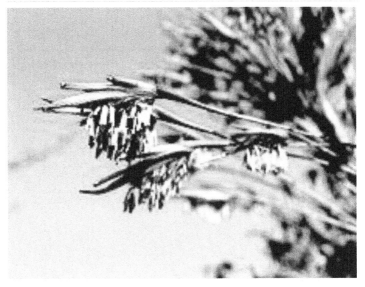

Flowering bamboo

Most bamboo species flower infrequently. In fact, many bamboos only flower at intervals as long as 65 or 120 years. These taxa exhibit mass flowering (or gregarious flowering), with all plants in a particular species flowering worldwide over a several year period. The longest mass flowering interval known is 130 years, and is found for all the species *Phyllostachys bambusoides* (Sieb. & Zucc.). In this species, all plants of the same stock flower at the same time, regardless of differences in geographic locations or climatic conditions, and then the bamboo dies. (Sounds like menopause kicking in at age 50 all over the world- no?) The lack of environmental impact on the time of flowering indicates the presence of some sort of "alarm clock" in each cell of the plant which signals the diversion of all energy to flower production and the cessation of vegetative growth. This mechanism, as well as the evolutionary cause behind it, is still largely a mystery. [*My note--if reproduction hormones that cause flowering and seed production also cause aging-the mystery is solved.*]

One theory to explain the evolution of this semelparous mass flowering is the predator satiation hypothesis. This theory argues that by fruiting at the same time, a population increases the survival rate of their seeds by flooding the area with fruit, so that even if predators eat their fill, there will still be seeds left over. By having a flowering cycle longer than the lifespan of the rodent predators, bamboos can regulate animal populations by causing starvation during the period between flowering events. Thus, according to this hypothesis, the death of the adult clone is due to resource exhaustion, as it would be more effective for parent plants to devote all resources to creating a large seed crop than to hold back energy for their own regeneration. (*My note--this is probably true, as I believe both sex and aging are evolved defenses to evolving predation, which I will describe in a subsequent book.*)

A second theory, the fire cycle hypothesis, argues that periodic flowering followed by death of the adult plants has evolved as a mechanism to create disturbance in the habitat, thus providing the seedlings with a gap in which to grow. This hypothesis argues that the dead culms create a large fuel load, and also a large target for lightning strikes, increasing the likelihood of wildfire. Because bamboos can be aggressive as early successional plants, the seedlings would be able to outstrip other plants and take over the space left by their parents.

However, both have been disputed for different reasons. The predator satiation theory does not explain why the flowering cycle is 10 times longer than the lifespan of the local rodents, something not predicted by the theory. *(My note-there might have been a longer living predator of bamboo that drove this life history which is now extinct!)* The bamboo fire cycle theory is considered by a few scientists to be unreasonable; they argue that fires only result from humans and there is no natural fire in India. This notion is considered wrong based on distribution of lightning strike data during the dry season throughout India. However, another argument against this theory is the lack of precedent for any living organism to harness something as unpredictable as lightning strikes to increase its chance of survival as part of natural evolutionary progress.

In any case, flowering produce masses of seeds, typically suspended from the ends of the branches. These seeds will give rise to a new generation of plants that may be identical in appearance to those that preceded the flowering, or they may also produce new cultivars with different characteristics, such as the presence or absence of striping or other changes in coloration of the culms. –end Wikipedia article

PLANTS DIE IN AUTUMN

Why do most annual plants die in the autumn? Larry D. Nooden and Susan L. Schreyer at the University of Michigan are studying a chemical "death signal" possibly a hormone which they have traced to plant seeds. The possibility is being considered that seeds inside mature fruits such as soybean pods send out hormones, which cause plants to yellow and die even before nights cold enough for freezing cut them down.

Gardeners for years have known that if faded flowers are picked before they form seeds the plants will continue to produce more flowers. Pansies are a good example. Among the vegetables, okra will continue from early spring to frost if the pods are kept picked before they harden.

Nooden says that this idea was tested on soybeans. Growing pods were plucked from one side of the plant only and allowed to remain on the other. The side with the mature pods and seeds turned yellow and died, the other remained healthy.

Now for my favorite obvious case of programmed aging-the Pacific Salmon!

This example is so threatening to the mainstream evolutionary biologists' view of the world and aging that they classify it as a separate form of aging that does not have anything to do with the rest of the animal kingdom. By hiding it in the special category "semalparous aging" they can conveniently ignore it and go on with their outrageous self-deception and flat-earth world view of aging as a non-programmed "accident" of evolution.

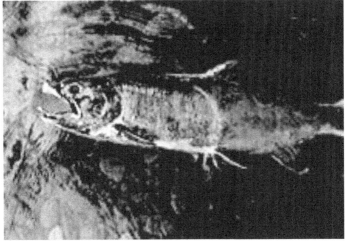

3 days after spawning

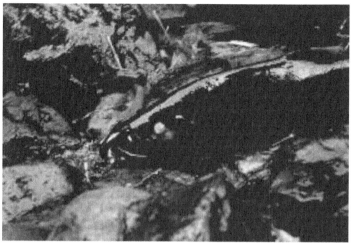
traveling upstream before spawning

All species of Pacific salmon (not including steelhead) die shortly after spawning. The one above was photographed at a spawning site along Eagle Creek in Oregon.

(From Wikipedia--**Semelparity** and **iteroparity** refer to the reproductive strategy of an organism. A species is considered *semelparous* if it is characterized by a single reproductive episode before death, and *iteroparous* if it is characterized by multiple reproductive cycles over the course of its lifetime.)

Well let's take a peak at "semelparous aging" in the Pacific Salmon, that grows up in an inland river on the Pacific side of the North American continent, and eventually travels down the river to live in the open sea for about 3 years.

After 3 years, the Salmon leave the oceans and swim back up the river in which they were born to return to the place of their birth. During this process, their reproductive hormones kick in at high gear and cause them to change and age rapidly. Once they reach their birthplace, they mate, lay their eggs, and then rapidly age and die within 3 days. If you castrate them, they can live much longer--up to 7 years. There is also an Atlantic Salmon that has a similar life history, except when infected with a parasite that has a 12-year life cycle, guess what? These salmon live 12 years instead of 3. So what is going on here?

It sounds to you and me like their reproductive hormones not only drive reproduction but also aging. But to mainstream aging theorists, the rigors of swimming upstream and the mating frenzy and resulting stress is what is killing these fish--not the act of reproduction and its associated hormones. There is a little logic to this, except for the fact that Alzheimer's has now been found to be driven by the sex-related hormone LH, which kind of puts the nail in their stress-aging theory coffin. The days of "accidental" aging are coming to a close. Unfortunately, our college professors don't realize it yet. They *really* don't like the furniture rearranged. Our amazing scientists will hear nothing of the Pacific Salmon. They prefer to plug their ears, shut their eyes and kick like little children, and banish this example of aging to a category they can ignore-- semelparous aging.

I am 100% sure that the Pacific Salmon is not an exception to aging in humans and mammals, but a great starting point for understanding aging and aging-related diseases in all animals.

Just for fun I will tell you about a study done by an aging researcher, Marc Tatar, from Brown University. He figured out how to manipulate the fruit fly larvae so that the development/reproduction related hormone called "juvenile hormone" (probably a fruit fly version of human LH) was not able to cause the larvae to develop. He did this by messing with their JH receptors somehow. He exposed these larvae to juvenile hormone for a while, and then later repaired their JH receptors with some sort of trick, and found that exposure to the Juvenile Hormone actually aged the flies and gave them shorter life span without causing them to develop. Thus, he proved that development/reproduction hormones also have a second function--to age the animal independently of development.

I saw him at an aging science conference and told him if I was in charge of the Nobel Prize, he should get 10 of them. "You just proved that aging is programmed and that means group selection is a real force of evolution." He looked at me like I had just farted! This is how blind scientists are to new thinking. They HATE IT. Ever since the biologist George Williams terribly ridiculed the idea of group selection in 1966. The army of our autistic scientists just repeated it like a mantra. Tatar had no idea of the importance of his discovery due to his being trapped in the logical box. Williams' thinking led to all the work and ridicule put out by Richard Dawkins on the "Selfish Gene." The funny thing is that the future will be ridiculing

Williams and Dawkins like they were Lamarckians. Lamarck predated Darwin, and suggested that giraffes grew (evolved) longer necks by the act of stretching to reach higher leaves. He is held up to ridicule now by our semi-autistic/pedantic scientists--but it turns out there actually *are* Lamarckian forms of evolution that occur through DNA imprinting.

Being locked in their logical boxes, our scientists and evolutionary theorists--geniuses that they are--still cannot explain the evolutionary purpose of sex, male and female sex types, and aging. One would think if they were working off the right theory these things would have been solved long ago. They just can't accept the idea that something that is bad for the spread of your genes could evolve because it is good for the group. They reject the idea of group selection--that an aging group of animals that reproduces sexually and has male and female sex types will outcompete a group of non aging animals that reproduce clonally. You see, they cannot understand why animals that engage in sex are only spreading half their genes, and not the 100% of their genes if they reproduced by cloning themselves. In their world, this does not compute. They've grabbed onto the "selfish gene" as the *only* driver of evolution. Thus, sex and aging do not make sense. In fact, a relatively recent issue of *Science* (our scientists' gospel-truth journal) was simply titled 'Sex," and the main thrust of the issue was that sex was still a theoretical mystery. By adhering to this belief that nothing bad for you could evolve and be selected for at the group level makes all our scientists completely blind to the idea that our "diseases of aging" are actually programmed into us, and are driven by hormones. The facts are coming out ahead of the theory. You will see a lot of egg on scientists' and theorists' faces in the near future. **If they could simply move past the logical boxes they are trapped in, it would be a simple matter to complete Darwin's theory of evolution which I will do in a subsequent book.**

To really make this idea most obvious, I will tell you about the type of animal that should exist everywhere if the idea that the selfish gene is the most important driver of evolution. That animal is known in academia as a *Darwinian Monster*. A Darwinian Monster starts reproducing right away after birth, reproduces asexually by just cloning itself, it never ages, has no reproductive decline, expands its numbers logarithmically, and eventually takes over all the spaces for living beings in the entire world. There are examples of animals who reproduce clonally, not needing sex (like some species of lizards), and there are examples of non-aging organisms that live 1000's of years (like the California Redwoods, Bristle Cone Pines, and Creosote bushes). But these are very rare. The bulk of living organisms defy the idea of the selfish gene being paramount by requiring the finding of a mate to reproduce, passing on only half their genes, having to live quite some time until reproductive maturity (puberty) is reached, then suffering from declining fertility and ultimately aging and death, which is the ultimate end to the spread of their genes. If the selfish gene theory were correct, the world would be dominated by Darwinian monsters, not by sexually reproducing, aging organisms. So for some reason, evolution does not want individuals to spread too many of their genes--and the mechanism as to how this happens is a bit more complicated than current scientists can figure out. So they continue to believe that the restraint of the spread of one's genes is impossible because they cannot imagine how it could happen. I say, **Think harder**--because it's obvious that gene restraint occurs.

Mainstream theorists are rabidly opposed to the idea that somehow evolution has created a way to limit the spread of an individual's genes by aging them, forcing them to find a mate to spread only ½ their genes per mating, and making individuals wait until puberty to reproduce. I find this rabid opposition quite similar to Creationists' suggestion that the very complex eye could never have evolved step-by-step from a simple eyespot because the eye is so complicated.

Creationists just don't have enough imagination to consider the idea of millions and millions of tiny improvements to the eye spot over many millions of years, eventually leading to a complex eye! Similarly, our eminent aging theory scientists seem to lack the insight to imagine scenarios where evolution can restrict the spread of genes by an individual for the good of the group.

Do we see semelparous aging in other animals? It is a bit rare, but it does exist in the marsupial male mice. Also, the female Octopus dies right after reproducing, allowing her young to consume her body.

The bottom-line common denominator in animals that die

immediately after reproducing is that their reproductive hormones not only drive reproduction but also drive the aging and programmed-death processes. Our scientists and theorists, trapped in their logical box will say it is impossible for a hormone that is bad for you to evolve.

If you start with the premise that reproductive hormones can kill salmon, annual plants, octopi, and marsupial mice, rather than hiding these examples of programmed aging in a category that can be ignored, you can easily transition to the idea that reproductive hormones also cause aging in "higher" animals like humans.

Thus we can then see the logic in why it might be possible that the human reproductive hormones of FSH and LH can also be the aging hormones that cause aging-related diseases and eventually kill you. The aging effects of FSH is a subject for another book--but let's just leave it at this-- LH attacks the body and causes atrophy of body parts, and cancers, when the atrophy does not occur as expected. (This occurs because the process of apoptosis [which is essentially cell suicide] occurs in the same way that cell reproduction occurs. It starts with separating the 2 DNA strands in our cells and removing any protections the DNA have from being copied. This also removes the protections from the DNA from being snipped into pieces and destroyed. When apoptosis goes right, it allows the DNA to be snipped up (instead of being copied), and the cell is destroyed. However, since apoptosis evolved from the same process that causes the cell to divide, when something goes awry, the cell reproduction process has been triggered but the DNA snipping process has been impaired, and you get *uncontrolled cell division*. Thus, instead of getting tissue atrophy, you get cancer).

LH also causes "little old-ladyism," since LH levels are way higher in females than males (you don't often hear of "little old men"). While FSH-caused aging occurs more often in males (due to FSH levels going way higher in males as a % of baseline vs. females), instead of destruction of tissue, it leads to the accumulation of tissue where it is not supposed to be. FSH does things for aging similar to stimulating follicles (or egg sacs (where they should not be) and leads to the "male diseases" of heart disease, hypertension, tissue calcification, and others. I'll leave it for another book--but FSH oddly is the only cAMP-stimulating hormone I have found that is not associated with cancer. (While LH is associated with almost all cancers!)_If there are any of you studying ahead of my next book, you will find it interesting that victims of the rapid aging disease of Progeria do not get cancer. I describe Progeria as an acceleration of the male diseases of aging. You might look at Progeria as what would happen if kids were born with super-bioactive FSH.

Here are some 12 year old kids with progeria (male and female):

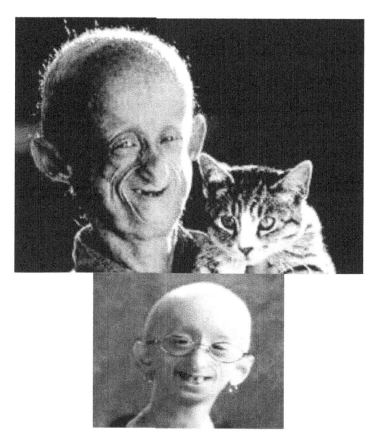

They sure look like old men no? I suggest they have

undergone an accelerated genetic version of the aging that is promoted by FSH (the primarily male aging hormone).

An interesting fact about progeria kids is that they are almost all quite smart (remember, men that hit age 90 are generally not demented, while women are?). And they don't get cancer, while other victims of rapid aging syndromes like Werner's syndrome (WS) which kicks in after puberty are often demented, and most get cancer.

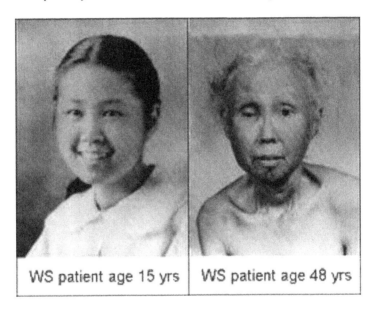

| WS patient age 15 yrs | WS patient age 48 yrs |

Werner's syndrome victims, I suggest, have undergone an accelerated genetic version of aging that is promoted by LH (the primarily female aging hormone).

Chapter Eight—Anti-Aging Effects of Caloric... and *Water* Restriction

The one protocol that all scientists concede that will dramatically slow the aging process is a regimen called caloric restriction, which has been known since Clive McKay's 1935 experiment where he dramatically increased the lifespan of young rats by feeding them only enough to survive, but not grow. He only gave them enough food to grow if they started to look like they were not thriving. Using this dietary regimen, he was able to increase their life spans by about 30-40% compared to rats that were fed all they wanted. What is not well known is that Clive McCay was a trout farmer, and accidentally noticed the same lifespan extension in his trout in the 1920's, when he went on vacation and his caretaker forgot to feed one group of fish which had to survive on any insects that fell in their tank. Both his trout observation and his rat experiment were published as papers in the *Journal of Nutrition,* I think around 1927 and 1935.

Our repetition-loving scientists have repeated this caloric restriction (CR) experiment over and over and over again. There are a huge number of CR experiments out there since McCay's 1935 paper--all saying the same thing--over and over and over--that *caloric restriction extends lifespan.* They even tried the experiment in monkeys at University of Wisconsin, and found--it works! It works in all animals tested, and it should work in humans. Yes we get it! You can stop now! The real question is, how does it work?

I'll get into this more later, but basically it boosts melatonin and DHEA levels in animals undergoing CR. There are probably other hormones affected that have not been tested. I know for sure that fasting (of at least 5 days) reduces LH and FSH dramatically in humans. (Note: if it finally is shown that CR does not increase the lifespan of monkeys or humans, it suggests to me that we apes have increased our lifespan as far as they can go without increasing the length of our telomeres which determine how many times our cells can divide.)

I asked myself in 1996, why does caloric restriction work from an evolutionary perspective? Does the lack of food in a famine slow the aging process to make sure any surviving animals will be "young" enough to reproduce once the famine is over? And does it prevent reproduction to prevent both the mother and the baby from dying instead of the lone female surviving? You see, starving animals lose the ability to reproduce until food returns (females more easily than males)--and they also *stop aging*! Can we make the simple leap that reproductive hormones (suppressed by famine) drive the aging process (which is suppressed by famine)?

Since 1935, our scientists and theorists have been repeating the caloric restriction experiment over and over. As of the year 2000 **I had only seen one** paper, published in the 1980's by Ed Masoro, where the idea was promoted that evolution slowed aging in a famine, and curtailed reproduction to maintain reproductive potential in the survivors so the group could survive. Having a baby in a famine decreases your odds of survival along with the baby's. That should give you an idea of how mentally handicapped our scientists are. Science moves way too slow because it is dominated by non-creative people who love repetition and sameness, and hate anything new.

Also around 1996, I asked myself--if famine leads to life extension in the animals involved, what causes famine? The answer was drought. Lack of water. Thus, I surmised, if lack of food slows the aging process to protect against famine, there should be a much stronger and longer life-extending effect caused by lack of water! Why? Because if a drought causes a famine, there will be plenty of dead plants and animals to eat during the early stages of the drought, so one that survives a drought will have lots of dehydrated food but very little water. Since the drought is longer than the famine, water restriction should increase lifespan longer than caloric restriction.

I then tested this idea in 10 rats--Sprague Dawley females. I repeated Clive McCay's experiment, except instead of withholding food to restrain growth, I withheld water. The rats could eat all the Doritos corn chips they wanted. To get a good survival curve for well-fed and well-watered rats, I used 8 rats as controls. I only had 2 water-restricted rats. So what happened?

Amazingly, one of my two water-restricted rats *lived longer than the longest living calorically restricted rats that I could find in all the experiments on the record*! It lived a *WORLD-record 47 months*. The oldest CR rat of this kind I could find lived 45 months, and there had been 1000's of this type of rat underwent caloric restriction (basically semi-starvation) to get their *one* long-liver of 45 months.

I have a little video on YouTube which you can see if you punch in http://youtu.be/skLVAQgWx60 in your browser. (You can also search for it by typing in "Longest living rat in the world" in the YouTube search box. It is posted by Jeffbo7777). I add this here just to demonstrate that I have had some luck in coming up with unusual, novel theories that make predictions that, when tested, are confirmed by the test results!

I told the head of the NIH's (the US Govt's National Institutes of Health) Methuselah Project (the Methuselah Project is inviting different experiment suggestions to create the longest lived mouse or rat, and then funding the most promising hoping it can be applied to human health) about my water restriction test results. Well, the head scientist (dingbat!) who runs the program said basically, "Oh that is interesting but we cannot do that experiment because dehydration is bad for you."

This "scientist" did not care that my rat had set an all-time record for lifespan. The idea of water restriction set off alarm bells in her head, since she had always been taught that *water is good for you*. This kind of proves a point that I will make later in this book about the sorry state of our science community today, run by semi-autistics who get mad if the furniture is rearranged.

One of my control rats got a huge solid tumor that I tried to cure by fasting. I withheld food until she lost almost 30% of her body weight. She went from about 290 grams to 220. It didn't work. My theory was that if your body is going to destroy and consume up to 30% of your cells due to starvation, that evolution would have programmed it to know to eat the tumor rather than your other critical tissues. I let her eat and get back to 280 grams, and fasted her again. No luck. So then I let her eat to get back to 280 again and then I water-fasted her, and Boom! The tumor which was the size of half a golf ball shrunk to the size of a penny and stayed there. And she was cured for 6 months. In human terms that would be about 20 years of remission. After 6 months, it blew up again. At this time, I had it biopsied just to make sure it was cancer, since my father, a Stanford-educated MD, told me it wasn't likely a tumor. But it was.

I gave these results to multiple scientists in the aging field, and they wanted nothing to do with them, and only tried to figure out why my water restriction experiment should be ignored. Eric LeBourg was the most dismissive. It was easy for them, since my experiment was done at home in a closet and not at a science lab, and I only had two experimental (water-restricted) animals. NEVER MIND THAT ONE OF THEM SET THE WORLD RECORD FOR LIFE SPAN FOR THE RAT TYPE IN QUESTION (SPRAGUE-DAWLEY FEMALES).

The one thing that scientists have found while studying caloric restriction (CR) in Rhesus monkeys at the University of Wisconsin is that CR causes the monkeys to have higher DHEA and melatonin levels than the controls. So this gives us a good idea of how melatonin is likely involved in slowing (or stopping) age-related diseases. (I will also add increased DHEA, as well as progesterone and pregnenolone as also preventing and stopping age-related diseases like Alzheimer's)

New Discovery May Safeguard Your Brain from Dementia
June 08 2012 |

By Dr. Mercola

Could fasting for two days a week prevent age-related brain shrinkage, heart disease, diabetes, and possibly even cancer? New research suggests that fasting triggers a variety of health-promoting hormonal and metabolic changes. Fasting - quantified as consuming somewhere between 500 and 800 calories in a day - has been shown to reduce:

- Growth factor - a hormone linked with cancer and diabetes
- "Bad" LDL cholesterol
- Cholesterol
- Inflammation levels

Overall, it also helps lessen damage from free radicals (dangerous molecules that cause damage in your body). Furthermore, according to the featured article in the Daily Mail[1]:

"Suddenly dropping your food intake dramatically... triggers protective processes in the brain... similar to the beneficial effect you get from exercise. This could help protect the brain against degenerative diseases such as Alzheimer's and Parkinson's."

Intermittent Fasting: A Good Alternative to Constant Calorie Restriction

While it's long been known that restricting calories in certain animals can increase their lifespan by as much as 50 percent, more recent research suggests that sudden and intermittent calorie restriction appears to provide the same health benefits as constant calorie restriction.

This is good news, as it may be easier to do for some people who cannot commit to chronically restrictive diet. The Daily Mail reports:

"Professor Mattson is one of the pioneers of research into fasting - a few years ago he made a breakthrough when he found rats could get nearly all the benefits of calorie restriction if the scientists only cut back their calories every other day.

On the next day the rats could eat as much as they liked and yet they showed the same benefits as rats on a low-calorie regimen all the time. Suddenly it looked as if humans could benefit from a form of calorie restriction regimen that, unlike daily restriction, is feasible to follow.

Now results of other trials are revealing the benefits.

In one study, reported last year in the International Journal of Obesity, a group of obese and overweight women was put on a diet of 1,500 calories a day while another group was put on a very low 500-calorie diet for two days, then 2,000 calories a day for the rest of the week. Both groups were eating a healthy Mediterranean-style diet. '

We found that both lost about the same amount of weight and both saw a similar drop in biomarkers that increase your risk of cancer,' says Dr Michelle Harvie, a dietitian at Manchester University who led the research.

'The aim was to find which was the most effective and we found that the women in the fasting group actually had a bigger improvement in sensitivity to insulin.' Improved insulin sensitivity means better control of blood sugar levels."

While I don't generally promote calorie restriction, it is an important piece of the puzzle, and this type of intermittent fasting may be helpful for many - especially in light of the compelling research supporting calorie restriction. Remember, fasting does not mean abstaining from ALL food, but rather a dramatic reduction of calorie intake.

You need to cut your daily calories at least in half, but can go as low as 500-800 calories a day. The KEY to successful calorie restriction, however, lies in *which calories* you cut, which I will review in a moment. But first, let's take a look at some of the health benefits of intermittent fasting.

The Surprising Health Benefits of Calorie Restriction

Interestingly, some of the mechanisms largely responsible for weight loss and diabetic control when fasting are also the ones responsible for the benefits to your brain. Research suggests that calorie restriction can protect brain cells and make them more resilient against stress. This protective effect is in part due to fasting's effect on leptin and ghrelin; two hormones involved in appetite regulation. According to Professor Mattson, these hormones are also involved in the process of renewing brain cells - especially in the hippocampus - *when you are not overweight.*

Your hippocampus is the area of your brain where most of your memory functions are located, and there's a strong relationship between the size of your hippocampus and memory performance.

According to the featured article[ii]:

"If you start putting on weight, levels of ghrelin drop and brain cell replacement slows. 'The effect is particularly damaging in your 40s and 50s, for reasons that aren't clear yet,' he [Professor Mattson] says. 'Obesity at that age is a marker for cognitive problems later.' The good news is that this brain-cell damage can be reversed by the two-day fasting regime, although so far Professor Mattson has shown this only in rats. A human trial is starting soon. There is reason to think it should work.

Fasting every other day had a striking effect on people with asthma in a small study he ran a few years ago. 'After eight weeks they had lost eight percent of their body weight, but they also benefited from the ability of calorie restriction to reduce inflammation. Tests showed that levels of inflammation markers had dropped by 90 per cent. As levels came down, their breathing became much easier,' says Professor Mattson."

There is one important caveat, however. Mattson's research showed that symptoms returned about two weeks after quitting the intermittent fasting, so it's really a lifestyle commitment, not a temporary fix. Some can handle intermittent fasting long-term whereas others might find it too challenging. Still, it's an option to consider if you're having health issues or weight problems.

Fasting and Exercise: Are They Compatible?

I've previously interviewed fitness expert Ori Hofmekler on the issue of fasting and exercise. According to Ori, fasting also has the surprising benefit of helping you reconstruct your muscles when combined with exercise. This is due to an ingenious preservation mechanism that protects your active muscle from wasting itself. In a nutshell, if you don't have sufficient fuel in your system when you exercise, your body will break down other tissues *but not the active muscle*, i.e. the muscle being exercised.

That said, neither Ori nor I advocate starvation combined with rigorous exercise. It's important to be sensible. And you need to consume sufficient amounts of protein in order to prevent muscle wasting. Also, while there's more science in support of calorie restriction than any other diet in the world today, there *are* side effects to chronic calorie restriction, such as decreased thyroid function and decreased testosterone.

In my own personal experimentation, I have definitely fasted too long and lost loads of muscle mass. So now I tend to use fasting if I have consumed foods that caused me to gain a few extra pounds. I will skip my breakfast and exercise fasting. My next meal will be lunch, and then I'll have dinner. This has worked quite well and allows me to easily drop a few pounds and get my body fat into the ideal range. It has worked so well that I am in the process of considering doing this on a permanent basis as it just makes loads of sense to replicate ancestral eating patterns that clearly did not have access to food 24/7,

Cut the Correct Calories...

One important fact that many tend to gloss over or ignore entirely when it comes to calorie restriction is *which type* of calories to restrict. From a biological standpoint, the important part is not really how many calories you eat per day; it's about getting the right nutrients. It's important to realize that all calories are NOT created equal, and will not have identical effects your weight or health. Their value depends on the types of food (nutrients) they're attached to.

In the US, six of the top 10 sources of calories are carbohydrates from sugars and grains[iii], and this is a major reason why so many Americans are overweight. They're simply eating far too many sugars. It's very important to restrict *carbs* when doing a calorie restrictive diet. Your body does not require sugars for optimal health, but it does require protein and fats.

When you cut out the sugars and carbs it is wise to replace them with high quality non-processed fats. Some of my favorites include organic grass-fed raw butter, eggs, coconut oil, avocados, and almonds.

There's very compelling evidence showing that calories from *fat* are far more beneficial for your health than calories from carbohydrates. And fear not... It's already been well established that stearic acid (found in cocoa and animal fat) has no effect on distorting your healthy cholesterol ratios at all, and actually gets converted in your liver into the monounsaturated fat called oleic acid. The other two, palmitic and lauric acid, *do* raise *total* cholesterol. However, since they raise "good" cholesterol as much or more than "bad" cholesterol, you're still actually *lowering* your risk of heart disease. And there are additional benefits.

Lauric acid (as from coconut oil) has shown to boost thyroid hormone activity along with the body's metabolic rate. This is obviously a huge advantage to those interested in weight loss or those who suffer from underactive thyroid.

I couldn't encourage you more to implement this program. It has radically improved my personal confidence in using diet choices to achieve high level wellness and optimal body fat. Cutting down on your grains and sugars, replacing them with high quality fats and skipping some meals, especially before exercise, seem to be a powerful combination to help you Take Control of Your Health.

References:

- The Daily Mail February 27, 2012
- The Daily Mail February 27, 2012
- Report of the Dietary Guidelines Advisory Committee on the Dietary Guidelines for Americans, 2010
- The Daily Mail February 27, 2012

Chapter Nine—LH Causes Alzheimer's--History of the Theory

In this chapter, I'll detail the development of the theory that LH is the cause of Alzheimer's disease. As I outlined in Chapter One, I was first struck by the almost universal rise of LH (and to a lesser degree, FSH) in Dilman and Dean's *Neuroendocrine Theory*, which was published in 1992 (based on Dilman's theory, which he first promulgated in a Ph.D. thesis in 1955). Although Dilman described in eloquent detail how the hypothalamic and neuroendocrine changes contributed to most age-related degenerative diseases, the subject of Alzheimer's disease was notable by its absence.

Let me show you the history of science articles that discuss LH *and* Alzheimer's (AD) in the same article. I searched PUB MED, the science article database that goes back to 1967, and has the vast majority of the modern world's scientific and medical studies and written by scientists to date. In this chapter, you will see there are 51 articles that mentioned LH and Alzheimer's in the same article. The oldest three mention LH and Alzheimer's only because they measured LH amongst various hormones. The 4th article in the chronology is mine, where I first suggest that LH *causes* AD. After that, there are many by Dr. Bowen, who *somehow* figured out the same crazy idea that LH causes AD--*right after my first paper*...Hmmmm! The papers are presented in *reverse order*, starting from the most recent (#1) to the oldest (# 51). Just browse through them, but notice the parts I highlighted or made comments on.

1. Phlorotannins from brown algae (Fucus vesiculosus) inhibited the formation of advanced glycation endproducts by scavenging reactive carbonyls. Liu H, Gu L. *J Agric Food Chem*. 2012 Feb 8;60(5):1326-34. Epub 2012 Jan 30.

2. Increased number of Purkinje cell dendritic swellings in essential tremor. Yu M, Ma K, Faust PL, Honig LS, Cortés E, Vonsattel JP, Louis ED. *Eur J Neurol*. 2012 Apr;19(4):625-630. doi: 10.1111/j.1468-1331.2011.03598.x. Epub 2011 Dec 5.

3. Direct exposure of guinea pig CNS to human luteinizing hormone increases cerebrospinal fluid and cerebral beta amyloid levels. Wahjoepramono EJ, Wijaya LK, Taddei K, Bates KA, Howard M, Martins G, deRuyck K, Matthews PM, Verdile G, Martins RN. *Neuroendocrinology*. 2011;94(4):313-22. Epub 2011 Oct 5.

4. Animal models for aberrations of gonadotropin action. Peltoketo H, Zhang FP, Rulli SB. *Rev Endocr Metab Disord*. 2011 Dec;12(4):245-58. Review.

5. Efficacy of voxel-based morphometry with DARTEL and standard registration as imaging biomarkers in Alzheimer's disease patients and cognitively normal

older adults at 3.0 Tesla MR imaging. Mak HK, Zhang Z, Yau KK, Zhang L, Chan Q, Chu LW. *J Alzheimers Dis.* 2011;23(4):655-64.

6. T1rho (T1ρ) MR imaging in Alzheimer's disease and Parkinson's disease with and without dementia. Haris M, Singh A, Cai K, Davatzikos C, Trojanowski JQ, Melhem ER, Clark CM, Borthakur A. *J Neurol.* 2011 Mar;258(3):380-5. Epub 2010 Oct 7.

7. Low luteinizing hormone enhances spatial memory and has protective effects on memory loss in rats. Ziegler SG, Thornton JE. *Horm Behav.* 2010 Nov;58(5):705-13. Epub 2010 Aug 5.

8. Investigation into the efficacy of the acetylcholinesterase inhibitor, donepezil, and novel procognitive agents to induce gamma oscillations in rat hippocampal slices. Spencer JP, Middleton LJ, Davies CH. *Neuropharmacology.* 2010 Nov;59(6):437-43. Epub 2010 Jun 23.

9. Disturbed sleep/wake rhythms and neuronal cell loss in lateral hypothalamus and retina of mice with a spontaneous deletion in the ubiquitin carboxyl-terminal hydrolase L1 gene. Pfeffer M, Plenzig S, Gispert S, Wada K, Korf HW, Von Gall C. *Neurobiol Aging.* 2012 Feb;33(2):393-403. Epub 2010 Apr 3.

10. Genetic ablation of luteinizing hormone receptor improves the amyloid pathology in a mouse model

of Alzheimer disease. Lin J, Li X, Yuan F, Lin L, Cook CL, Rao ChV, Lei Z. *J Neuropathol Exp Neurol.* 2010 Mar;69(3):253-61.

11. Augmented axonal defects and synaptic degenerative changes in female GRK5 deficient mice. Li L, Rasul I, Liu J, Zhao B, Tang R, Premont RT, Suo WZ. *Brain Res Bull.* 2009 Mar 16;78(4-5):145-51. Epub 2008 Oct 26.

12. Luteinizing hormone levels are positively correlated with plasma amyloid-beta protein levels in elderly men. Verdile G, Yeap BB, Clarnette RM, Dhaliwal S, Burkhardt MS, Chubb SA, De Ruyck K, Rodrigues M, Mehta PD, Foster JK, Bruce DG, Martins RN. *J Alzheimers Dis.* 2008 Jun;14(2):201-8.

13. Aging cebidae. Williams L. *Interdiscip Top Gerontol.* 2008;36:49-61. Review.

14. Characterization of a CNS penetrant, selective M1 muscarinic receptor agonist, 77-**LH**-28-1. Langmead CJ, Austin NE, Branch CL, Brown JT, Buchanan KA, Davies CH, Forbes IT, Fry VA, Hagan JJ, Herdon HJ, Jones GA, Jeggo R, Kew JN, Mazzali A, Melarange R, Patel N, Pardoe J, Randall AD, Roberts C, Roopun A, Starr KR, Teriakidis A, Wood MD, Whittington M, Wu Z, Watson J. *Br J Pharmacol.* 2008 Jul;154(5):1104-15. Epub 2008 May 5.

15. A luteinizing hormone receptor intronic variant is significantly associated with decreased risk of **Alzheimer's**

disease in males carrying an apolipoprotein E epsilon4 allele. Haasl RJ, Ahmadi MR, Meethal SV, Gleason CE, Johnson SC, Asthana S, **Bowen RL**, Atwood CS. *BMC Med Genet.* 2008 Apr 25;9:37.

16. Human chorionic gonadotropin (a luteinizing hormone homologue) decreases spatial memory and increases brain amyloid-beta levels in female rats. Berry A, Tomidokoro Y, Ghiso J, Thornton J. *Horm Behav.* 2008 Jun;54(1):143-52. Epub 2008 Mar 10.

17. Androgens in the etiology of **Alzheimer's disease** in aging men and possible therapeutic interventions. Fuller SJ, Tan RS, Martins RN. *J Alzheimers Dis.* 2007 Sep;12(2):129-42. Review.

18. Increases in luteinizing hormone are associated with declines in cognitive performance. Casadesus G, Milliken EL, Webber KM, **Bowen RL**, Lei Z, Rao CV, Perry G, Keri RA, Smith MA. *Mol Cell Endocrinol.* 2007 Apr 15;269(1-2):107-11. Epub 2007 Feb 6.

19. Human neurons express type I GnRH receptor and respond to GnRH I by increasing luteinizing hormone expression. Wilson AC, Salamat MS, Haasl RJ, Roche KM, Karande A, Meethal SV, Terasawa E, **Bowen RL**, Atwood CS. *J Endocrinol.* 2006 Dec;191(3):651-63.

20. Activation of estrogen receptor alpha increases and estrogen receptor beta decreases apolipoprotein E expression in hippocampus in vitro and in vivo. Wang JM,

Irwin RW, Brinton RD. *Proc Natl Acad Sci U S A*. 2006 Nov 7;103(45):16983-8. Epub 2006 Oct 31.

21. Steroidogenic acute regulatory protein (StAR): evidence of gonadotropin-induced steroidogenesis in **Alzheimer disease**. Webber KM, Stocco DM, Casadesus G, **Bowen RL**, Atwood CS, Previll LA, Harris PL, Zhu X, Perry G, Smith MA. *Mol Neurodegener*. 2006 Oct 3;1:14.

22. The role of gonadotropins in **Alzheimer's disease**: potential neurodegenerative mechanisms. Barron AM, Verdile G, Martins RN. *Endocrine*. 2006 Apr;29(2):257-69. Review.

23. The estrogen myth: potential use of gonadotropin-releasing hormone agonists for the treatment of **Alzheimer's disease**. Casadesus G, Garrett MR, Webber KM, Hartzler AW, Atwood CS, Perry G, **Bowen RL**, Smith MA. *Drugs R D*. 2006;7(3):187-93. Review.

24. Hormones and dementia - a comparative study of hormonal impairment in post-menopausal women, with and without dementia. Robusto-Leitao O, Ferreira H. *Neuropsychiatr Dis Treat*. 2006 Jun;2(2):199-206.

25. Transcription factor NF-kappaB: a sensor for smoke and stress signals. Ahn KS, Aggarwal BB. *Ann N Y Acad Sci*. 2005 Nov;1056:218-33. Review.

26. Beta-secretase (BACE1) inhibitors from Sanguisorbae Radix. Lee HJ, Seong YH, Bae KH, Kwon SH, Kwak HM,

Nho SK, Kim KA, Hur JM, Lee KB, Kang YH, Song KS. *Arch Pharm Res*. 2005 Jul;28(7):799-803.

27. The gonadotropin connection in **Alzheimer's disease**. Meethal SV, Smith MA, **Bowen RL**, Atwood CS. *Endocrine*. 2005 Apr;26(3):317-26. Review.

28. Serum estradiol, progesterone, testosterone, FSH and **LH** levels in postmenopausal women with **Alzheimer's** dementia. Tsolaki M, Grammaticos P, Karanasou C, Balaris V, Kapoukranidou D, Kalpidis I, Petsanis K, Dedousi E. *Hell J Nucl Med*. 2005 Jan-Apr;8(1):39-42.

29. Apolipoprotein E epsilon4 and catechol-O-methyltransferase alleles in autopsy-proven Parkinson's **disease**: relationship to dementia and hallucinations. Camicioli R, Rajput A, Rajput M, Reece C, Payami H, Hao C, Rajput A. *Mov Disord*. 2005 Aug;20(8):989-94.

30. Coordination modes between copper(II) and N-acetylneuraminic (sialic) acid from a 2D-simulation analysis of EPR spectra. Implications for copper mediation of sialoglycoconjugate chemistry relevant to human biology. Fainerman-Melnikova M, Szabó-Plánka T, Rockenbauer A, Codd R. *Inorg Chem*. 2005 Apr 4;44(7):2531-43.

31. Evidence for the role of gonadotropin hormones in the development of **Alzheimer disease**. Casadesus G, Atwood

CS, Zhu X, Hartzler AW, Webber KM, Perry G, **Bowen RL**, Smith MA. *Cell Mol Life Sci.* 2005 Feb;62(3):293-8. Review.

32. Low free testosterone is an independent risk factor for **Alzheimer's disease**. Hogervorst E, Bandelow S, Combrinck M, Smith AD. *Exp Gerontol.* 2004 Nov-Dec;39(11-12):1633-9.

33. Mitochondrial complex I inhibition depletes plasma testosterone in the rotenone model of Parkinson's **disease**. Alam M, Schmidt WJ. *Physiol Behav.* 2004 Dec 15;83(3):395-400.

34. Beyond estrogen: targeting gonadotropin hormones in the treatment of **Alzheimer's disease**. Casadesus G, Zhu X, Atwood CS, Webber KM, Perry G, **Bowen RL**, Smith MA. *Curr Drug Targets CNS Neurol Disord.* 2004 Aug;3(4):281-5. Review.

35. Gonadotropin-induced gene regulation in human granulosa cells obtained from IVF patients: modulation of genes coding for growth factors and their receptors and genes involved in cancer and other diseases. Rimon E, Sasson R, Dantes A, Land-Bracha A, Amsterdam A. *Int J Oncol.* 2004 May;24(5):1325-38.

36. [Spectral analysis of EEG coherence in **Alzheimer's disease**]. Calderón González PL, Parra Rodríguez MA, Llibre Rodríguez JJ, Gutiérrez JV. *Rev Neurol.* 2004 Mar 1-15;38(5):422-7. Spanish.

37. **Bowens next paper** Luteinizing hormone, a reproductive regulator that modulates the processing of amyloid-beta precursor protein and amyloid-beta deposition. **Bowen RL**, Verdile G, Liu T, Parlow AF, Perry G, Smith MA, Martins RN, Atwood CS. *J Biol Chem.* 2004 May 7;279(19):20539-45. Epub 2004 Feb 9.

38. Elevated sex-hormone binding globulin in elderly women with **Alzheimer's disease**. Hoskin EK, Tang MX, Manly JJ, Mayeux R. *Neurobiol Aging.* 2004 Feb;25(2):141-7.

39. Vascular pathology in **Alzheimer disease**: correlation of cerebral amyloid angiopathy and arteriosclerosis/lipohyalinosis with cognitive decline. Thal DR, Ghebremedhin E, Orantes M, Wiestler OD. *J Neuropathol Exp Neurol.* 2003 Dec;62(12):1287-301.

40. Relationship between testosterone, sex hormone binding globulin and plasma amyloid beta peptide 40 in older men with subjective memory loss or dementia. Gillett MJ, Martins RN, Clarnette RM, Chubb SA, Bruce DG, Yeap BB. *J Alzheimers Dis.* 2003 Aug;5(4):267-9.

41. Testosterone and gonadotropin levels in men with dementia. Hogervorst E, Combrinck M, Smith AD. *Neuro Endocrinol Lett.* 2003 Jun-Aug;24(3-4):203-8.

42. Multiple luteinizing hormone receptor (LHR) protein variants, interspecies reactivity of anti-LHR mAb clone

3B5, subcellular localization of LHR in human placenta, pelvic floor and brain, and possible role for LHR in the development of abnormal pregnancy, pelvic floor disorders and **Alzheimer's disease.** Bukovsky A, Indrapichate K, Fujiwara H, Cekanova M, Ayala ME, Dominguez R, Caudle MR, Wimalsena J, Elder RF, Copas P, Foster JS, Fernando RI, Henley DC, Upadhyaya NB. *Reprod Biol Endocrinol.* 2003 Jun 3;1:46.

43 **Every year Bowen seems to be pumping out a new paper! Now he has picked up Craig Atwood as his co-researcher.** Elevated luteinizing hormone expression colocalizes with neurons vulnerable to **Alzheimer's disease** pathology. **Bowen RL**, Smith MA, Harris PL, Kubat Z, Martins RN, Castellani RJ, Perry G, Atwood CS. J Neurosci Res. 2002 Nov 1;70(3):514-8.

44. [Normal and pathologic implication of cytokines]. Stratone A, Stratone C, Chiruță R, Topoliceanu F. Rev Med Chir Soc Med Nat Iasi. 2001 Oct-Dec;105(4):657-61. Review. Romanian.

45. **Bowen is on a roll!** Elevated gonadotropin levels in patients with **Alzheimer disease.** Short RA, **Bowen RL**, O'Brien PC, Graff-Radford NR. *Mayo Clin Proc.* 2001 Sep;76(9):906-9.

(>>>>>**Then, out of the blue--Dr. Bowen has an amazing insight!~!**<<<<<)

46. An association of elevated serum gonadotropin concentrations and Alzheimer disease? **Bowen RL,** Isley JP, **Atkinson RL.** *J Neuroendocrinol.* 2000 Apr;12(4):351 -4.

47. Gonadal function in young women with Down syndrome. **NO LINK SUGESTED** Angelopoulou N, Souftas V, Sakadamis A, Matziari C, Papmeletiou V, Mandroukas K. *Int J Gynaecol Obstet.* 1999 Oct;67(1):15-21.

*******(first mention ever of an LH/AD connection in this paper) *******
48. The evolution of aging: a new approach to an old problem of biology. Bowles JT. *Med Hypotheses.* **1998 Sep;51(3):179-221.**

-**Until my paper AD and LH had only been mentioned together in these 3 papers since 1967!! And no one suggested a link!**

49 .Pharmacokinetics of MDL 26479, a novel benzodiazepine inverse agonist, in normal volunteers. **NO AD/LH LINK SUGGESTED** Robbins DK, Hutcheson SJ, Miller TD, Green VI, Bhargava VO, Weir SJ. *Biopharm Drug Dispos.* 1997 May;18(4):325-34.

50. [Neuroendocrinological aspects of aging]. **NO AD/LH LINK SUGGESTED** Vermeulen A. *Verh K Acad Geneeskd Belg.* 1994;56(4):267-80. Dutch.

51. Pressor, norepinephrine, and pituitary responses to two TRH doses in **Alzheimer's disease** and normal older men. **NO AD/LH LiNK SUGGGESTED** Lampe TH, Veith RC, Plymate SR, Risse SC, Kopeikin H, Cubberley L, Raskind MA. *Psychoneuroendocrinology.* 1989;14(4):311-20.

Here is the full abstract from my 1998 paper:

Med Hypotheses. 1998 Sep;51(3):179-221.

The evolution of aging: a new approach to an old problem of biology.

Bowles JT.

JeffBo AT aol DOT com

Abstract

Most gerontologists believe aging did not evolve, is accidental, and is unrelated to development. The opposite viewpoint is most likely correct. Genetic drift occurs in finite populations and leads to homozygosity in multiple-alleled traits. Episodic selection events will alter random drift towards homozygosity in alleles that increase fitness with respect to the selection event. Aging increases population turnover, which accelerates the benefit of genetic drift. This advantage of aging led to the evolution of aging systems (ASs). Periodic predation was the most prevalent episodic selection pressure in evolution. Effective defenses to predation that allow exceptionally long lifespans to evolve are shells, extreme intelligence, isolation, and flight. Without episodic predation, aging provides no advantage and aging systems will be deactivated to increase reproductive potential in unrestricted environments. The periodic advantage of aging led to the periodic evolution of aging systems. Newer aging systems co-opted and added to prior aging systems. Aging organisms should have one dominant, aging system that co-opts vestiges of earlier-evolved systems as well as vestiges of prior systems. In human evolution, aging systems chronologically emerged as follows: telomere shortening, mitochondrial aging, mutation accumulation, senescent gene expression (AS#4), targeted somatic tissue apoptotic-atrophy (AS#5), and female reproductive tissue apoptotic-atrophy (AS#6). During famine or drought, to avoid extinction, reproduction is curtailed and aging is slowed or somewhat reversed to postpone or reverse reproductive senescence. AS#4-AS#6 are gradual and reversible aging systems. The life-extending/rejuvenating effects of caloric restriction support the idea of aging reversibility. Development and aging are timed by the gradual loss of cytosine methylation in the genome. Methylated cytosines (5mC) inhibit gene transcription, and deoxyribonucleic acid (DNA) cleavage by restriction enzymes. Cleavage inhibition prevents apoptosis, which requires DNA fragmentation. Free radicals catalyze the demethylation of 5mC while antioxidants catalyze the remethylation of cytosine by altering the activity of DNA methyltransferases. Hormones act as either surrogate free radicals by stimulating the cyclic adenosine monophosphate (cAMP) pathway or as surrogate antioxidants through cyclic guanosine monophosphate (cGMP) pathway stimulation. Access to DNA containing 5mC inhibited developmental and aging genes and restriction sites is allowed by DNA helicase strand separation. Tightly wound DNA does not allow this access. The DNA helicase generates free radicals during strand separation; hormones either amplify or counteract this effect. Caloric restriction slows or reverses the aging process by increasing melatonin levels, which suppresses reproductive and free radical hormones, while increasing antioxidant hormone levels. Cell apoptosis during CR leads to somatic wasting and a release of DNA, which increases bioavailable cGMP. The rapid aging diseases of progeria, the three diseases: (xeroderma pigmentosum (XP), Cockayne syndrome(CS), and ataxia telangiectasia (AT)), and Werner's syndrome are related to or caused by defects in three separate DNA helicases. The rapid aging diseases caused by mitochondrial malfunctions mirror those seen in XP, CS, and AT. Comparing these diseases allows for assignment of the different symptoms of aging to their respective aging systems. Follicle-stimulating hormone (FSH) demethylates the genes of AS#4, luteinizing hormone (LH) of AS#5, and estrogen of AS#6 while cortisol may act cooperatively with FSH and LH, and 5-alpha dihydrotestosterone (DHT) with FSH in these role. The Werner's DNA helicase links timing of the age of puberty, menopause, and maximum lifespan in one mechanism. Telomerase is under hormonal control. Most cancers likely result from malfunctions in the programmed apoptosis of AS#5 and AS#6. The Hayflick limit is reached primarily through loss of cytosine methylation of genes that inhibit replication. Men suffer the diseases of AS#4 at a higher rate than women who suffer from AS#5 more often. Adult mammal cloning suggests aging-related cellular demethylation, and thus aging, is reversible. **This theory suggests that the protective effect of smoking and ibuprofen for Alzheimer's disease is caused through LH suppression**.

Now, here is the actual excerpt from my paper where I develop the LH/AD link:

Unsolved mysteries:

The many paradoxes of cigarette smoking

The model of human aging that has been developed so far apparently is a bit simplistic as it does not adequately explain the many paradoxes of cigarette smoking. Exceptions have been found to be exciting markers of areas that require further research to gain an even further understanding of the aging process.

Nicotine and cigarette smoking have been shown to cause major endocrine changes in humans. The majority of the literature suggests that smoking reduces (or does not affect) estrogen but increases testosterone in women, while not affecting testosterone and increasing estrogen in men. In both sexes, increased cortisol, and vasopressin levels are observed as well as a decrease in LH. (**185a, 185b, 186**). The well known increase in lung cancer may be explained by vasopressin as high levels of vasopressin have been implicated in being potentially involved in inducing lung cancer (**187**). If the contact of smoke with the lugs was the primary cause of lung cancer, then one might expect to see high incidences of lung cancer in marijuana smokers which is apparently not the case. Also, the gender differences in smoking's effects on sex hormones seems to be consistent with the cortisol-related inhibition of fertility mentioned earlier.

Cigarette smoking is well known to be associated with increasing the risks of myocardial infarction (**188**), and may be involved in accelerating hair loss, hair graying, and facial wrinkling, all symptoms of AS#4 (**189**) This occurs without any apparent smoking-induced increase in FSH, but can be explained if cortisol, as earlier proposed, can act cooperatively with FSH to demethylate the aging genes of AS#4.

The interesting paradoxes are found in that smoking seems to confer a protective effect against Alzheimer's (AD) , Parkinson's disease (PD) and Tourette's Syndrome which all likely belong to AS#5 (**190**), and seems to protect against uterine and endometrial cancer in women (**191**), while not increasing the incidence of breast cancer (**192**). Much of this makes sense in that reduced LH should lead to inhibiting the brain atrophy of AS#5, and a reduction in estrogen should lead to an inhibition of the cancers of sex tissues of AS#6.

Additional weight is given to the LH/Alzheimer's connection by the recently publicized suggestion that ibuprofen administration reduces the risk of Alzheimer's after two studies were found through a Medline search that show that ibuprofen suppresses LH (**198, 199a**).

Here is a table from my aging paper that suggests which hormones drive which forms of aging. The important columns are for FSH and LH

Aging System #4 Senescent Gene Expression: FSH/DHT driven, seen in men at higher rate. (co-opts #3) (and #1?)	Aging System #5A Somatic atrophy: Mitochondrial Apoptosis, LH/hCG driven, seen in women at a higher rate (co-opts #2)	Aging System #5B Somatic atrophy: nDNA Fragmentation Apoptosis, LH/hCG driven, seen in women at a higher rate	Aging System # 6 Sex tissue atrophy: estrogen/DHT driven, seen in women at higher rate (co-opts #4, #5, (and #1))
Progeria only. Defective DNA helicase type #1.	Mitochondrial Myopathy (MM), NARP (N), CPEO (CP), MELAS (ME), MERRF (MR) , KSS (K), Dystonia (D), Leigh's Syndrome (LS)	Ataxia Telangiectasia (AT), Xeroderma Pigmentosum (XP), Cockayne Syndrome (CS). Defective DNA helicase type #2.	Werner's Syndrome. (WS), Bloom's Syndrome (BS), Defective DNA helicase type #3.
Original to #4 alone (likely defects of development)			
Coxa Valga & necrosis of head of femur			
Dysplastic osteoporosis			
Symptoms of #4 co-opted by #6			Symptoms of #6 co-opted from #4
Atherosclerosis			Atherosclerosis-WS
Hypertension			Hypertension-WS
Gray Hair			Gray Hair-WS
Alopecia			Alopecia-WS
Calcification of Heart Valves			Calc. of Heart Valves-WS
Laryngeal Atrophy			Laryngeal Atrophy-WS
Loss of subcutaneous tissue			Loss of subcut. tissue-WS
Hypermelanosis of			Hypermelanosis of

Skin			Skin-WS
Hypogonadism (defect of development?)		Hypogonadism - AT, XP	Hypogonadism -WS, BS
	Symptoms of #5A also seen in #5B and co-opted by #6	Symptoms of #5B also seen in #5A and co-opted by #6	Symptoms of #6 co-opted from #5A and #5B
	Muscle Wasting-MM, N	Muscle Wasting-AT	Muscle Wasting-WS
	Neuronal Degeneration/Brain Atrophy-CP, ME, MR, K	Neuronal Degeneration/Brain Atrophy -AT, XT	Neuronal Degeneration, Brain Atrophy -WS
	Basal Ganglion Calcification - D, LS	Basal Ganglion Calcification - CS	Basal Ganglion Calcification -WS
	Cataracts-K	Cataracts-CS	Cataracts-WS
	Diabetes-K	Diabetes-AT	Diabetes-BS, WS
	Alzheimer's Disease-mitochondrial induced	Alzheimer's Disease-XP	Alzheimer's Disease-WS
		Symptoms of #5B co-opted by #6	Symptoms of #6 co-opted from #5B
		Poor Healing -XP	Poor Healing -WS
		Skin Ulcers -XP	Skin Ulcers -WS
		Thymic Atrophy-AT	Thymic Atrophy-BS, WS
		Scaly Skin-XP	Scaly Skin-WS
		Somatic Cancers-XP,AT	Somatic Cancers-BS, WS
		Lipofuscin Accumulation-CS,XP	Lipofuscin Accumulation-WS
		Arthritis-AT	Arthritis-WS
		Peripheral Osteoporosis-CS	Peripheral Osteoporosis-WS
			Symptoms unique to #6
			Menopause-WS
			Breast, Uterine, and Ovarian atrophy and cancer-WS
			Prostate atrophy-WS, hyperplasia-

More from my paper:

Some hormone levels change significantly in humans with age.

Several hormones that are proposed free radical surrogates _increase_ with age, and in some cases, dramatically.

In human males:
-Estradiol increases from about 125 pmol/liter at age 45 to about 265 pmol per liter by age 80, more than a 200% increase **(30).**
-**LH** starts in a range of about 1.0 to 2.8 ml.U./mL at age 40 and increases to a range of 2.1 to 11 ml. U./mL by age 80: anywhere from a 60% to 1100% increase **(31).**
-**FSH** at age 50 begins at about 2.5 ml.U./mL and increases to a range of 6 to 50 ml.U./mL by age 80: a 140% to 2000% increase. **(the maximum % increase in range from baseline exceeds that in females) (32).**

In human females,
-**LH** increases from a range of 5 to 45 mU/mL at age 40 to a range of 40 to 130 mU/mL by age 55, a change of anywhere from flat to +2600%. **(the maximum % increase in range from baseline exceeds that in males) (33)**
-FSH increases in women from about 20 ml.U./mL at the age of 40 to anywhere from 40 to 200 ml. U./mL by age

75.....a 100% to 1000% percent increase **(combined values from 31, 33).**
-Estrogen and its related hormones increase quite significantly around the time of menopause and then, unlike the males' sustained rise, crash precipitously when menopause is complete. **(34).**

Likewise, we see many antioxidant surrogate hormones _declining_ dramatically with age

In human males:
-Testosterone typically ranges in males from about 3.5 to 10.5 ng/mL at age 40 and declines to a range of .4 to 4 ng/mL by age 80 **(35).**
-DHEA declines from about 3600 ng/mL at age 20 to about 800 ng/mL by age 70 **(36)**

In human females:
-Testosterone levels are reported to decline by 50% from age 21 to age 40 **(37).**
-DHEA declines from about 2600 ng/mL a age 20 to about 800 ng/mL by age 70 **(38)**

In both sexes:
-Peak melatonin levels (which occur at night) in the elderly are 50% less than those of young adults while basal melatonin levels remain constant. **(39).**
-Peak growth hormone levels (which occur at night) are reported to be diminished or completely absent in some subjects over 50 years of age and decline from as high as 2.9 ng/mL to 1.1 ng/mL **(40).**

One last thing from my paper:

Melatonin: the famine and drought hormone.

During famine conditions or CR one would expect that in addition to the increase in cGMP activity, that an increase in cGMP stimulating hormones would be seen. Also, one would expect a decline in cAMP stimulating hormones. In a study of human males undergoing 5 days of fasting (**136**) the following hormone level changes were seen, (for hormones not measured in this study other references are noted):

cAMP stimulating hormones:
TSH declined by 67%-as expected
LH decreased by 33%-as expected
FSH decreased by 33%-as expected
Cortisol increased by 110%-unexpected
Estrogen -increased by 10%-unexpected

cGMP stimulating hormones
Melatonin increased +/-100% in rats (**137**)-as expected
GH increased 200%-400% in men (**138**) -as expected
DHEA-S increased 100%-expected
Testosterone-decreased 50%- unexpected

T3 and T4 were relatively unaffected, and prolactin declined 25% but is not listed because it is an "ambidextrous" hormone stimulating both cAMP and cGMP depending on which receptors it influences.

The above results reasonably conform to expectations based on the prior hypothesis regarding cAMP and cGMP stimulating hormones. However, by examining the exceptions additional important insights can be gained. First, the cortisol increase of 110% is definitely not expected as it is a cAMP hormone and the hormone is widely known to be implicated in accelerating the diseases of aging in persons where it is chronically elevated. What is also known about cortisol is that it has been implicated in triggering apoptosis is various cell types including thymocytes of the thymus gland (139). If the early stages of CR require a large scale induction of apoptosis in various cells, it is likely that the increased cortisol is involved. The other contradiction about the large cortisol increase is that when it occurs during CR one must assume that it does not lead to the deleterious accelerated age changes that are normally associated with high cortisol levels as CR'd animals live much longer than controls. One study explains the contradiction: during CR, although the baseline levels of cortisol are elevated, increases in peak cortisol levels from stress are shown to be lower in CR'd animals than in ad lib fed animals (140). The idea that evolution has designed stress so that at times it kills and at other times it does not suggests that stress is also an aging system. This idea will be explored shortly.

The other exceptions include a 10% increase in estrogen and a 50% decrease in testosterone. If one remembers that inhibition of reproduction would be a primary goal of the CR response, then a drop in the male reproductive hormone is not illogical even though it is a cGMP hormone. The corresponding increase in DHEA of 100% which in absolute terms is of equal magnitude to the testosterone decline might be seen as CR's version of testosterone that does not induce sexuality in the male. Finally, if the only male aging symptoms associated with AS#6 include prostatic atrophy (assuming no malfunctions in apoptosis) then the estrogen increase of 10% can also be seen as an anti-reproductive hormone change. An estrogen increase however, would not be expected to occur in the female during CR, and studies show that this is likely true (**141**).

CR leads to quite a complicated array of hormone changes, but can it all be simplified? A simple Medline search of **melatonin** against each of the individual hormones mentioned above provides the answer. Melatonin administration has been shown to suppress LH (**142**), FSH (**143**), and testosterone (**144**) while increasing DHEA (**145**), GH (**146**), and in some cases cortisol (**147**) levels in either rats, mice or humans. In females, 300 mg. of melatonin was shown to suppress estrogen (E2) levels (**148**). More definitive studies do need to be made in this area, however, as most studies are short term in nature while melatonin induced hormone changes seem to take much longer to occur in humans. Melatonin's effect on prolactin, however, was not clear and is generally suggestive of increasing levels in humans but this might only be a short term effect due to the short term nature of human melatonin studies. Melatonin, did however, reduce prolactin levels in the rat pituitary (**149**). TSH was also shown to be suppressed in the rat by melatonin. (**150**) In most cases of hormone changes induced by CR, melatonin administration induced the same effect. What is also interesting, a reduction in body temperature in animals is seen during CR and posited by some to be the potential candidate as the active life-extending mechanism in CR. As one would expect, melatonin administration leads to reduced body temperature as well (**151a**). It is interesting to note that water deprivation, as would be expected, has also been shown to increase melatonin levels in rodents (**151b**).

And finally here is an abstract from a 2010 paper put out by a top scientist (Wang) at the United States National Institutes of Health (NIH)

Gonadotropin-releasing hormone receptor system: modulatory role in aging and neurodegeneration. Wang L, Chadwick W, Park SS, Zhou Y, Silver N, Martin B, Maudsley S. *CNS Neurol Disord Drug Targets*. 2010 Nov;9(5):651-60

Receptor Pharmacology Unit, National Institute on Aging, National Institutes of Health, Biomedical Research Center, Baltimore MD 21224, USA.

Abstract
Receptors for hormones of the hypothalamic-pituitary-gonadal axis are expressed throughout the brain. Age-related decline in gonadal reproductive hormones cause imbalances of this axis and many hormones in this axis have been functionally linked to neurodegenerative pathophysiology. Gonadotropin-releasing hormone (GnRH) plays a vital role in both central and peripheral reproductive regulation. GnRH has historically been known as a pituitary hormone; however, in the past few years, interest has been raised in GnRH actions at non-pituitary peripheral targets. GnRH ligands and receptors are found throughout the brain where they may act to control multiple higher functions such as learning and memory function and feeding behavior. The actions of GnRH in mammals are mediated by the activation of a unique rhodopsin-like G

protein-coupled receptor that does not possess a cytoplasmic carboxyl terminal sequence. Activation of this receptor appears to mediate a wide variety of signaling mechanisms that show diversity in different tissues. Epidemiological support for a role of GnRH in central functions is evidenced by a reduction in neurodegenerative disease after GnRH agonist therapy. It has previously been considered that these effects were not via direct GnRH action in the brain, however recent data has pointed to a direct central action of these ligands outside the pituitary. We have therefore summarized the evidence supporting a central direct role of GnRH ligands and receptors in controlling central nervous physiology and pathophysiology.

NIH News: New paper suggests elevated LH behind AD

This is a very well referenced and comprehensive review of the literature and data surrounding the concepts of elevated GNRH/LH contributing to AD. Probably most important, it was conducted and prepared by one of the leading neuroscientists at the NIH. Completely independent and with no ties to any private company. Gonadotropin-releasing hormone receptor system: modulatory role in aging and ...

Reply 1: NIH News!!! New paper suggests elevated LH behind AD
onward replied
"These findings support the premise that GnRH receptor-based therapeutics could be a potential therapeutic target for the treatment of AD. Several double-blind placebo controlled phase II clinical trials are currently underway to conclusively make this determination." Very interesting and encouraging. Thanks for posting, Prodiver. Can anyone find out exactly what "GnRH receptor-based therapeutics...

Reply 2: NIH News!!! New paper suggests elevated LH behind AD
Billstrailrunning replied
These findings support the premise that GnRH receptor-based therapeutics could be a potential therapeutic target for the treatment of AD. Several double-blind placebo controlled phase II clinical trials are currently underway

This sounds promising. We will look forward to the results of the intervention. Not sure what the intervention will be and will it be the same or different for males and ...

Reply 3: NIH News!!! New paper suggests elevated LH behind AD
Prodiver replied
Leuprolide acetate is the compound under study in the <u>Phase II</u> B trials. It is formulated in a patented biopolymer implant, developed by DURECT Corporation. According to the company, it uniquely releases a proprietary dosage level which is much higher than is used in previous applications of the compound to treat prostate cancer, endomitriosis or precocious puberty. LA has been shown to be very ...

Reply 4: NIH News!!! New paper suggests elevated LH behind AD
Billstrailrunning replied
Hey ProDiver, great research on your part. I have to say though I'm not thrilled at giving my ADLO <u>Lupron</u>. It is heavy on side-effects. Here is a link: http://www.drugs.com/sfx/leuprolide-side-effects.html.
That said, if there is even a hint that it really works I definitely would consider it for my ADLO. Male patients prescribed this medicine are fighting prostate cancer and those I have met are...

Appendices

Appendix A: melatonin treatment on secretion of steroid hormones

Am J Vet 2011 May;72(5):675-80.

Effect of combined lignan phytoestrogen and melatonin treatment on secretion of steroid hormones by adrenal carcinoma cells.

Fecteau KA, Eiler H, Oliver JW

Department of Comparative Medicine, College of Veterinary Medicine, University of Tennessee, Knoxville, TN 37996, USA. kfecteau@utk.edu

Abstract

OBJECTIVE: To investigate the in vitro effect of the combination of lignan enterolactone (ENL) or lignan enterodiol (END) withmelatonin on steroid hormone secretion and cellular aromatase content in human adrenal carcinoma cells.

SAMPLE: Human adrenocortical carcinoma cells.

PROCEDURES: Melatonin plus ENL or END was added to cell culture medium along with cAMP (100µM); control cells received cAMP alone. Medium and cell lysates were collected after 24 and 48 hours of cultivation. Samples of medium were analyzed for progesterone, 17-hydroxyprogesterone, androstenedione, aldosterone, estradiol, and cortisol concentration by use of radioimmunoassays. Cell lysates were used for western blot analysis of aromatase content.

RESULTS: The addition of ENL or END with melatonin to cAMP-stimulated cells (treated cells) resulted in significant decreases in estradiol, androstenedione, and cortisol concentrations at 24 and 48 hours, compared with concentrations in cells stimulated with cAMP alone (cAMP control cells). The addition of these compounds to cAMP-stimulated cells also resulted in higher progesterone and 17-hydroxyprogesterone concentrations than in cAMP control cells; aldosterone concentration was not affected by treatments. Compared with the content in cAMP control cells, aromatase content in treated cells was significantly lower.

CONCLUSIONS AND CLINICAL RELEVANCE: The combination of lignan and melatonin affected steroid hormone secretion by acting directly on adrenal tumor cells. Results supported the concept that this combination may yield similar effects on steroid hormone secretion by the adrenal glands in dogs with typical and atypical hyperadrenocorticism.
PMID: 21529220 [PubMed - indexed for MEDLINE]

Appendix B: Two twins with Alzheimer's

J Pineal Res 1998:25:260-263

Two twins with Alzheimer's and one takes melatonin: A

case report

Brusco LL, Marquez M, Cardinali DP. Monozygotic twins with Alzheimer's disease treated with melatonin: case report. J. Pineal Res. 1998; 25:260-263. @ Munksgaard, Copenhagen
Departamente of Fisiologie and Cultadde Medicina
Universidad de Buenos Aires,
Argentina

Abstract: Monozygotic twins with Alzheimer's disease of 3 years duration were studied. The onset of the disease differed by about 6 months between twins and was characterized by a primary impairment of memory function. Clinical evaluation at the time of diagnosis indicated a similar cognitive and neuroimaging alteration in both patients, as well as a similar neuropsychological impairment. A possible genetic origin of the disease was suggested as similar diseases suffered by the mother. Patients were initially treated with vitamin E (800 iu/day|. starting at approximately the same time (about 3 years ago), they received 50 mg/day thioridazine because of the behavioral and sleep disorder. One of the patients was treated with melatonin (6 mg orally) at bed time daily for 36 months. Evolution of the disease in the melatonin-treated patient indicated a milder impairment of memory function, with substantial improvement of sleep quality and reduction of sundowning. This led to discontinuance after 3 months of thioridazine treatment. Present clinical evaluation indicated a difference in functional stage of the disease between the twins (Functional Assessment Tool For

Alzheimer's Disease (FAST), with a score of 5 in the twin who received melatonin and of 7b in the twin who did not receive it. Since experimental data on melatonin in Animals indicated its antioxidant, antiapoptotic, and B-amyloid-decreasing activity, the hypothesis that melatonin has a beneficial effect in Alzheimer's disease patients should be considered.

Alzheimer's disease (AD) shows familial and sporadic forms, and several genetic defects have been identified that chiefly explain early-onset familial cases. Although most cases are sporadic, half the patients with sporadic AD have a positive family history. The mode of genetic transmission and the role of environmental factors are unknown (Breitner and Murphy, 1992; Small et al., 1993; Raiha et al., 1996; Bergeme ral.,1997; Gatz et al.,1997; Selkoe, 1997; Steffens et al.,1991). Monozygotic and dizygotic twins in later adulthood have been studied to examine genetic and environmental contributions to the decline of cognitive performance and eventually to the development of AD. The twin method for investigating genetic and environmental causes of disease has been applied mostly in early-onset illnesses. Analysis of late-on-set disorders like AD, requires examination.

Common assumptions about the relation between genetic causes and the degree of concordance expected. Several epidemiological studies have shown the Existence of a genetic etiology in some cases of AD. Pedigrees with an increased incidence of AD have been described in the literature. Some of these contain sufficient numbers of affected individuals in multiple generations to provide a rigorous argument for an autosomal dominant inheritance of the AD phenotype (Brcitner and Murphy, 1992; Bergem et al., 1991; Garz et al.,1997).

In recent years the possible therapeutic relevance of melatonin in AD have been suspected (Reiter, 1995). Melatonin protects neurons against B-amyloid toxicity and inhibits amyloid formation. (Pierpaoli, et al., 1998], B-amyloid-induced lipid peroxidation [Daniels et al., 1998], alters the metabolism of the B-amyloid precursor protein (Song and Lahiri, 1997), and prevents the oxidative damage by B-amyloid of mitochondrial DNA (Pozner et al., 1997). The probability of an absent melatonin rhythm is higher in demented patients compared with subjects without dementia (Fuchida et al., 1995). Moreover, we recently reported that treatment with melatonin of dementia patients having sleep disorders resulted in a significant improvement of "sundowning," namely, episodes of agitated behavior that are more severe at night and are found in most AD patients (Feinstein et al., 1997).

Since the study of monozygotic twins could be useful to elucidate possible therapeutic actions of melatonin in genetically identical subjects, we hereby report evolution of AD in a pair of monozygotic male twins, one of whom was treated with melatonin.

Case report
Two79-yearld male monozygotic twins with AD diagnosed 8 years earlier were studied. The onset of the disease

differed by about 6 months between both twins. The two patients have lived at their homes with their spouses, who have been the caretakers. They lived in closely similar environments, their standard of living being that corresponding to the middle class and with very similar family support conditions. The patients did not have any other organic disorder, alcohol abuse, or heavy smoking habits. Neuropsychological evaluation at diagnosis indicated a primary impairment of memory function in both twins. Both patients had similar cognitive and neuroimaging alterations, as well as a similar neuropsychological impairment at diagnosis. NMR at the time of diagnosis indicated the existence of a bi-temporal atrophy to a similar extent in both patients. A possible genetic origin of the disease was suggested by the fact that the mother suffered from AD.

Patients were initially treated with vitamin E (800 I.U./day). Starting at approximately the same time (about 3 years in advance to present assessment). They received in addition 50 mg/day thioridazine because of the behavioral and sleep disorder. Patient N.N. was treated with melatonin (3 mg gelatin capsules, Melatonin, Elisium S.A., Buenos Aires). In a dose of 6 mg orally at bed-time daily for 36 months. Three months after starting melatonin treatment, patient N.N. discontinued thioridazine and remained on a combined prescription of melatonin (6 mg/day) plus vitamin E (80C l.U./day) until present assessment.

At the time of present assessment a neuropsychological

evaluation of twins by the Functional Assessment Tool for Alzheimer's Disease (FAST) (Bauer and Reisberg, 1997) indicated a differential progression of the disease. Patient Z.Z. showed a 7b stage in FAST (e.g., inability to control the elimination of urine or feces; comprehension of single words only), whereas patient N.N. was in a 5 stage (e.g., inability to undertake complex tasks like financial planning or planning a meal; reluctance to comply with hygienic rules). Impairment of memory function was severe for patient Z.Z. while patient N.N. showed a milder picture (score 0/30 and 10/30 in the Mini-Mental-test, respectively). NMR at the time of present assessment showed a generalized cortical atrophy in both patients, with a more important bi-temporal atrophy and ventricular enlargement in patient Z.Z. (Fig. I).

In the neurologic exam, patient Z.Z. showed impaired walking and the presence of primitive reflexes (palmar prension, hyper-metamorphosis, and suckling reflex). He did not exhibit signs of focalization nor was he at a high risk for vasculopathy, as shown by a Flachinski scale= 1 (Flachinski et al., 1975). Pacing in patient Z.Z. was intense and increased at the evening; he was an insomniac and exhibited sundowning episodes. Speech ability of patient Z.Z. was severely impaired, being unable to pronounce or to understand simple words.

A very different clinical picture was found for patient N.N. In the neurologic exam, he showed normal walking and only rudiments of primitive reflexes (sucking reflex). Speech ability of patient N.N. was only slightly impaired and remained at approximately a similar degree for the last 3 years. Sleep-vigilance rhythm in patient N.N. was unimpaired. As his brother, he did not exhibit signs of focalization nor was he at risk for vasculopathy (Flachinski scale= 1).

Overall, patient N.N. exhibited lack of progression of the cognitive and behavioral signs of the disease, as evaluated clinically, during the time he received melatonin. In contrast, patient Z.Z. showed a significant deterioration of clinical conditions of the disease, with pacing, sleep disorders, loss of speech abilities, psychomotor agitation, and presence of primitive reflexes.

Discussion
The differential evolution of AD in the pair of monozygotic twins either receiving or not melatonin described herein is presumably ascribed to melatonin treatment. Such a putative therapeutic activity of melatonin in AD is not without sound experimental basis, since melatonin was reported to interfere in vitro with B-amyloid-related processes (Pozner et al., 1997; Pierpaoli, et al, 1997, 1998; Song and Lahiri, 1997; Daniels et al., 1998).

Appendix C: Alzheimer's Disease—Clinical Stages

Alzheimer's Disease—Clinical Stages

The Stages of Alzheimer's Disease	
At the New York University Medical Center's Aging and Dementia Research Center, Barry Reisberg, MD and colleagues have developed the Functional Assessment Staging (FAST) scale, which allows professionals and caregivers to chart the decline of people with Alzheimer's disease. The FAST scale has 16 stages and sub-stages:	
FAST Scale Stage	**Characteristics**
1... normal adult	No functional decline.
2... normal older adult	Personal awareness of some functional decline.
3... early Alzheimer's	Noticeable deficits in

disease	demanding job situations.
4... mild Alzheimer's	Requires assistance in complicated tasks such as handling finances, planning parties, etc.
5... moderate Alzheimer's	Requires assistance in choosing proper attire.
6... moderately severe Alzheimer's	Requires assistance dressing, bathing, and toileting. Experiences urinary and fecal incontinence.
7... severe Alzheimer's	Speech ability declines to about a half-dozen intelligible words. Progressive loss of abilities to walk, sit up, smile, and hold head up.

Detailed Description of Each of the 7 Stages

Stage 1 No cognitive decline. No subjective complaints of memory deficit. No memory deficit evident on clinical interviews.

Stage 2 (Forgetfulness)

163

Very mild cognitive decline. Subjective complaints of memory deficit, most frequently in the following area:

forgetting where one has placed familiar objects;

forgetting names formerly knew well.

No objective evidence of memory deficit on clinical interview. No objective deficits in employment or social situations. Appropriate concern regarding symptoms.

Stage 3
(Early Confusional)
Mild cognitive decline. Earliest clear-cut deficits. Manifestations in more than one of the following areas:

patient may have gotten lost when traveling to an unfamiliar location;

co-workers become aware of patient's relatively low

performance;
word and name finding
deficit becomes
evident to intimates;
patient may read a
passage of a book and
retain relatively little
material;
patient may demonstrate
decreased facility in
remembering names
upon introduction to
new people;
patient may have lost or
misplaced an object of
value;
concentration deficit may
be evident on clinical
testing.
Objective evidence of
memory deficit obtained
only with an intensive
interview. Denial begins to
become manifest in patient.
Mild to moderate anxiety
accompanies symptoms.

Stage 4
(Late Confusional)
Moderate cognitive decline.
Clear-cut deficit on careful

clinical interview.
Deficit manifest in following areas:

decreased knowledge of current and recent events;

may exhibit some deficit in memory of one's personal history;

concentration deficit elicited on serial subtractions;

decreased ability to travel, handle finances, etc.

Frequently no deficit in the following areas:

orientation to time and person;

recognition of familiar persons and faces;

ability to travel to familiar locations.

Inability to perform complex tasks. Denial is dominant defense mechanism. Flattening of affect and withdrawal from challenging situations occur.

Stage 5
(Early Dementia)
Moderately severe cognitive decline. Patient can no longer survive without some assistance. Patient is unable during interview to recall a major relevant aspect of their current lives, e.g., an address or telephone number of many years, the names of close family members (such as grandchildren), the name of the high school or college from which they graduated. Frequently some disorientation to time (date, day of week, season, etc.) or to place. An educated person may have difficulty counting back from 40 by 4s or from 20 by 2s. Persons at this stage retain knowledge of many major facts regarding themselves and others. They invariably know their own names and generally know their spouse' and children's

names. They require no assistance with toileting and eating, but may have some difficulty choosing the proper clothing to wear.

Stage 6
(Middle Dementia)
Severe cognitive decline. May occasionally forget the name of the spouse upon whom they are entirely dependent for survival. Will be largely unaware of all recent events and experiences in their lives. Retain some knowledge of their past lives but this is very sketchy. Generally unaware of their surroundings, the year, the season, etc. May have difficulty counting from 10, both backward and sometimes forward. Will require some assistance with activities of daily living, e.g., may become incontinent, will require travel assistance but occasionally will display

ability to familiar locations. Diurnal rhythm frequently disturbed. Almost always recall their own name. Frequently continue to be able to distinguish familiar from unfamiliar persons in their environment.
Personality and emotional changes occur. These are quite variable and include:
delusional behavior, e.g., patients may accuse their spouse of being an impostor, may talk to imaginary figures in the environment, or to their own reflection in the mirror;
obsessive symptoms, e.g., person may continually repeat simple cleaning activities;
anxiety agitation, and even previously nonexistent violent behavior may occur;
cognitive abulla, i.e., loss of willpower because an individual cannot

carry a thought long enough to determine a purposeful course of action. **Stage 7 (Late Dementia)** Very severe cognitive decline. All verbal abilities are lost. Frequently there is no speech at all - only grunting. Incontinent of urine, requires assistance toileting and feeding. Lose basic psychomotor skills, e.g., ability to walk, sitting and head control. The brain appears to no longer be able to tell the body what to do. Generalized and cortical neurologic signs and symptoms are frequently present. **Alzheimer's Disease and Skill Abilities** Dr Reisberg has also shown that the decline typical of Alzheimer's disease is the flip side of normal skill acquisition by infants, children, and young adults:	
Ability	**Age of acquisition**

	during normal development	
Hold a job. Function independently in the world.	12 years and older	
Handle simple finances.	8-12 years	
Select proper clothing.	5-7 years	

Apppendix D: Smoking Prevents Alzheimer's

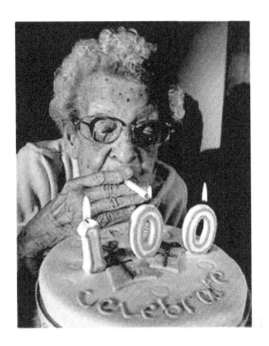

By Mike

WASHINGTON, D.C., July 21, 2011–An exhaustive 20 year study conducted by Washington Roast Investigators and the American Scientific Society has conclusively concluded that smoking cigarettes prevents the devastating advance of Alzheimer's dementia (AD). In fact the study shows that the more you smoke the less likely you are to develop the brain clogging tangles and plaques of AD. The study, financed by Phillip Morris, followed thousands of smokers over a 20 year period and found that few if any developed the disease. Theories range anywhere from a change in the blood supply to brain neurons to a chemical in tobacco that blocks plaque development. Critics on the other side contend that chain smokers die before they get Alzheimer's.

Forces International   *THERAPEUTIC EFFECTS OF SMOKING AND NICOTINE*

Smoking lowers Parkinson's disease risk - More evidence that smoking fights Parkinson - "A new study adds to the previously reported evidence that cigarette smoking protects against Parkinson's disease. Specifically, the new research shows a temporal relationship between smoking and reduced risk of Parkinson's disease. That is, the protective effect wanes after smokers quit."

Impact of Smoking on Clinical and Angiographic Restenosis After Percutaneous Coronary Intervention– This large study shows yet another benefit of smoking. This time the benefit concerns restenosis, that is, the occlusion of coronary arteries. Smokers have much better chances to survive, heal and do well. Where is the press? Nowhere to be found, of course; we are talking about a significant positive about tobacco and smoking, which affects the health of people, don't we? Well, **come on!** We are also talking about *responsible media*, here... people better increase their chances of death from cardiovascular disease then *getting the idea that smoking may be good for them* – a totally unacceptable paradox.

The Oxford English Dictionary defines paradox in

these terms: "*A statement or tenet contrary to received opinion or belief ... as being discordant with what is held to be established truth, and hence absurd or fantastic*". Since the benefits of smoking are too numerous and consistent to be attributable to error or random chance, it follows that the *established truth asserting that smoking is the cause of (almost) all disease cannot be true* – a reality that dramatically clashes with the gigantic corruption of public health, its pharmaceutical and insurance mentors, institutions and media. Therefore, it is constantly suppressed in the interest of public health, but not of the people.

Twin Study Supports Protective Effect of Smoking For Parkinson's Disease – *"Dr. Tanner's group continued to see significant differences when dose was calculated until 10 years or 20 years prior to diagnosis. They conclude that this finding refutes the suggestion that individuals who smoke more are less likely to have PD because those who develop symptoms quit smoking." "'The inverse association of smoking dose and PD can be attributed to environmental, and not genetic, causes with near certainty," the authors write.'*

Total silence from the antismoking mass media droids, of course, on this pivotal, long-range study that shows yet another benefit of smoking. The reasons are obvious, and they need no further comments. If the intention of "public health" is to inform the public about the consequences of smoking on health as it proclaims, why don't we see "warnings" such as: **"Smoking Protects against Parkinson's Disease,"** or **"Smoking protects against Alzheimer's Disease,"** or **"Smoking protects against Ulcerative Colitis"** and so on, alongside with the other speculations on "tobacco-related" disease? Isn't the function of public health to tell the citizens about ALL the effects on health of a substance? Obviously not. "Public health," today, is nothing more than a deceiving propaganda machine paid by pharmaceutical and public money to promote frauds, fears, and puritanical rhetoric dressed up in white coats.

Does tobacco smoke prevent atopic disorders? A study of two generations of Swedish residents- *"In a multivariate analysis, children of mothers who smoked at least 15 cigarettes a day tended to have lower odds for suffering from allergic rhino-conjunctivitis, allergic asthma, atopic eczema and food allergy, compared to children of mothers who had never smoked (ORs 0.6-0.7). Children of fathers who had smoked at least 15 cigarettes a day had a similar tendency (ORs 0.7-0.9)."*

Kids of smokers have LOWER asthma! You certainly won't see this one on the health news of BBC or ABC, as they are too busy trying to convince us that smokers "cause" asthma in their kids - and in the kids of others. That, of course, is not true, as smoking does not "cause" asthma.

Shocker: 'Villain' nicotine slays TB - *"Nicotine might* *be a surprising alternative someday for treating stubborn forms of tuberculosis, a University of Central Florida researcher said Monday. The compound stopped the growth of tuberculosis in laboratory tests, even when used in small quantities, said Saleh Naser, an associate professor of microbiology and molecular biology at UCF. ... Most scientists agree that nicotine is the substance that causes people to become addicted to cigarettes and other tobacco products."*

"... But no one is suggesting that people with TB take up the potentially deadly habit of smoking." Of course not. It is much better to develop medication-resistant superbugs than to start smoking...It should be said that the "most scientists" in question are paid off by the pharmaceutical industry for their research; and that most of the aforementioned "scientists" promote the nicotine-based "cessation" products manufactured by their masters -- mysteriously without explaining **why** such an addictive substance becomes ***"un-addictive"*** when used *to quit smoking!*

Carbon Monoxide May Alleviate Heart Attacks And Stroke Carbon monoxide is a by-product of tobacco smoke. A report indicates very low levels of carbon monoxide may help victims of heart attacks and strokes. Carbon monoxide inhibits blood clotting, thereby dissolving harmful clots in the arteries. The researchers focused on carbon monoxide's close resemblance to nitric oxide which keeps blood vessels from dilating and prevents the buildup of white blood cells. *"Recently nitric oxide has been elevated from a common air pollutant . . . to an [internal] second messenger of utmost physiological importance. Therefore, many of us may not be entirely surprised to learn that carbon monoxide can paradoxically rescue the lung from [cardiovascular blockage] injury."* The pharmacological benefits of tobacco are nothing new.

Smoking Prevents Rare Skin Cancer - A researcher at the National Cancer Institute is treading treacherous waters by suggesting that smoking may act as a preventative for developing a skin cancer that primarily afflicts elderly men in Mediterranean regions of Southern Italy, Greece and Israel. Not that smoking should be recommended for that population, Dr. James Goedert is quick to assure his peers. What is important is not that smoking tobacco may help to prevent a rare form of cancer but that there is an admission by a researcher at the National Cancer Institute that there are ANY benefits to smoking.

Smoking Reduces The Risk Of Breast Cancer - A new study in the *Journal of the National Cancer Institute* (May 20, 1998) reports that carriers of a particular gene mutation (which predisposes the carrier to breast cancer) who smoked cigarettes for more than 4 pack years (i.e., number of packs per day multiplied by the number of years of smoking) were found to have a statistically significant 54 percent decrease in breast cancer incidence when compared with carriers who never smoked. One strength of the study is that the reduction in incidence exceeds the 50 percent threshold.

However, we think it important to point out that this was a small, case control study (only 300 cases) based on self-reported data.

Nitric oxide mediates a therapeutic effect of nicotine in ulcerative colitis - *"CONCLUSIONS: Nicotine reduces circular muscle activity, predominantly through the release of nitric oxide-this appears to be 'up-regulated' in active ulcerative colitis. These findings may explain some of the therapeutic benefit from nicotine (and smoking) in ulcerative colitis and may account for the colonic motor dysfunction in active disease."*

Effects of Transdermal Nicotine on Cognitive Performance in Down's Syndrome - *"We investigated the effect of nicotine-agonistic stimulation with 5 mg transdermal patches, compared with placebo, on cognitive performance in five adults with the disorder. Improvements possibly related to attention and information processing were seen for Down's syndrome patients compared with healthy controls. Our preliminary findings are encouraging..."*

More benefits of nicotine. Of course, it is politically incorrect to say that this is a benefit of *smoking* - only of the pharmaceutically-produced transdermal nicotine, the one that is terribly addictive if delivered through cigarettes, but not addictive at all, and even *beneficial*, when delivered through patches.... Antismoking nonsense aside, nicotine gets into the body regardless of the means of delivery. And more evidence about the benefits seems to emerge quite often, though the small size of this study cannot certainly be taken as conclusive.

Nicotine Benefits- The benefits of nicotine -- and smoking -- are described in this bibliography. This information is an example of what the anti-tobacco groups do not want publicized because it fails to support their agenda. Some of the studies report benefits not just from nicotine, but from *smoking itself.* But of course, according to the anti-smokers, all these scientists have been "paid by the tobacco industry" ... even though this is not true. Sadly, personal slander and misinformation are the price a scientist has to pay for honest work on tobacco.

Parkinson's Disease Is Associated With Non-smoking - Bibliography of references from studies associating Parkinson's disease with non-smoking. Certain benefits of smoking are well-documented, but the anti-smoking groups, backed by several medical journals (more interested in advertising revenue than in informing the population), are silent. By the way, what about the *cost of non-smokers to society due to their prevailing tendency to contract Parkinson's disease?*

Alzheimer's Disease Is Associated With Non-Smoking - *"A statistically significant inverse relation between smoking and Alzheimer's disease was observed at all levels of analysis, with a trend towards decreasing risk with increasing consumption".*

Research indicating that nicotine holds potential for

non-surgical heart by-pass procedures honored by the American college of cardiology - Dr. Christopher Heeschen of Stanford University was honored by the American College of Cardiology for his research on the effect of nicotine on angiogenesis (new blood vessel growth). His work took third place in the 2,000 entry Young Investigators Competition in the category of Physiology, Pharmacology and Pathology. Dr. Heeschen presented compelling data from research done at Stanford revealing that the simple plant protein, nicotine, applied in small harmless doses, produced new blood vessel growth around blocked arteries to oxygen-starved tissue.

Smoking Your Way to Good Health - The benefits of smoking tobacco have been common knowledge for centuries. From sharpening mental acuity to maintaining optimal weight, the relatively small risks of smoking have always been outweighed by the substantial improvement to mental and physical health. Hysterical attacks on tobacco notwithstanding, smokers always weigh the good against the bad and puff away or quit according to their personal preferences.

Now the same anti-tobacco enterprise that has spent billions demonizing the pleasure of smoking is providing additional reasons to smoke. Alzheimer's, Parkinson's, Tourette's Syndrome, even schizophrenia and cocaine addiction are disorders that are alleviated by tobacco. Add in the still inconclusive indication that tobacco helps to prevent colon and prostate cancer and the endorsement for smoking tobacco by the medical establishment is good news for smokers and non-smokers alike. Of course the revelation that tobacco is good for you is ruined by the pharmaceutical industry's plan to substitute the natural and relatively inexpensive tobacco plant with their overpriced and ineffective nicotine substitutions. Still, when all is said and done, the positive revelations regarding tobacco are very good reasons indeed to keep lighting those cigarettes.

Does maternal smoking hinder mother-child transmission of Helicobacter pylori infection? - *"Evidence for early childhood as the critical period of Helicobacter pylori infection and for clustering of the infection within families suggests a major role of intrafamilial transmission. In a previous study, we found a strong inverse relation between maternal smoking and H. pylori infection among preschool children, suggesting the possibility that mother-child transmission of the infection may be less efficient if the mother smokes. To evaluate this hypothesis further, we carried out a subsequent population-based study in which H. pylori infection was measured by 13C-urea breath test in 947 preschool children and their mothers. We obtained detailed information on potential risk factors for infection, including maternal smoking, by standardized questionnaires. Overall, 9.8% (93 of 947) of the children and 34.7% (329 of 947) of the mothers were infected. Prevalence of infection was much lower among children of uninfected mothers (1.9%) than among children of infected mothers (24.7%). There was* *a strong inverse relation of children's infection with maternal smoking (adjusted odds ratio = 0.24; 95% confidence interval = 0.12-0.49) among children of infected mothers, but not among children of uninfected mothers. These results support the hypothesis of a predominant role for mother-child transmission of H. pylori infection, which may be less efficient if the mother smokes. ".*

Risk of papillary thyroid cancer in women in relation to smoking and alcohol consumption. - *"Both smoking and alcohol consumption may influence thyroid function, although the nature of these relations is not well understood. We examined the influence of tobacco and alcohol use on risk of papillary thyroid cancer in a population-based case-control study. Of 558 women with thyroid cancer diagnosed during 1988-1994 identified as eligible, 468 (83.9%) were interviewed; this analysis was restricted to women with papillary histology (N = 410). Controls (N = 574) were identified by random digit dialing, with a response proportion of 73.6%. We used logistic regression to calculate odds ratios (OR) and associated confidence intervals (CI) estimating the relative risk of papillary thyroid cancer associated with cigarette smoking and alcohol consumption. A history of ever having smoked more than 100 cigarettes was associated with a reduced risk of disease. This reduction in risk was most evident in current smokers.*

Women who reported that they had ever consumed 12

or more alcohol-containing drinks within a year were also at reduced risk (OR 0.7, 95% CI = 0.5-1.0).
Similar to the association noted with smoking, the reduction in risk was primarily present among current alcohol consumers. The associations we observed, if not due to chance, may be related to actions of cigarette smoking and alcohol consumption that reduce thyroid cell proliferation through effects on thyroid stimulating hormone, estrogen, or other mechanisms. "

Urinary Cotinine Concentration Confirms the Reduced Risk of Preeclampsia with Tobacco Exposure- This study, though small, shows one of the benefits of smoking during pregnancy. *"These findings, obtained by using laboratory assay, confirm the reduced risk of developing preeclampsia with tobacco exposure. (Am J Obstet Gynecol 1999;181:1192-6.) "*

Fact Sheet on Smoking and Alzheimer's- From Forest UK.

Smokers have reduced risks of Alzheimer's and Parkinson's disease- Of the 19 studies, 15 found a reduce risk in smokers, and none found an increased risk. And smoking is clearly associated with a reduced risk of Parkinson's disease, another disease in which nicotine receptors are reduced. The fact that acute administration of nicotine improves attention and information processing in AD patients adds further plausibility to the hypothesis.

The Puzzling Association between Smoking and Hypertension during Pregnancy- This large study has examined nearly 10,000 pregnant women. Conclusion: *"Smoking is associated with a reduced risk of hypertension during pregnancy. The protective effect appears to continue even after cessation of smoking. Further basic research on this issue is warranted. (Am J Obstet Gynecol 1999;181:1407-13.)*

Smoking: Protection Against Neural Tube Defects? - Swedish researchers have some surprising news for pregnant women who smoke: a decreased risk of neural tube defects in babies.

Smoking Linked to Alzheimer's and Dementia

Study Shows Heavy Smoking between Ages 50 and 60 May Raise Risk of Alzheimer's Disease
By Bill Hendrick
WebMD Health News
Reviewed by Laura J. Martin, MD

Oct. 25, 2010 -- People who are heavy smokers in their midlife years are more than doubling their risk of developing Alzheimer's disease or other forms of dementia two decades later, a new study shows.

While smoking has long been known to increase the risk of dying from cancer and heart disease, researchers in Finland say they've found strong reason to believe that smoking more than two packs of cigarettes daily from age 50 to 60 increases risk of dementia later in life.

Scientists at the University of Eastern Finland and at Kuopio University Hospital, Finland, analyzed data from 21,123 members of a health care system who took part in a survey between 1978 and 1985, when they were between ages 50 and 60.

Diagnoses of dementia, Alzheimer's disease, and vascular dementia were tracked from Jan. 1, 1994, when participants were 71.6 years old, on average, through July 31, 2008.

Among the key findings:

- 25.4% of the participants, or 5,367 people, were diagnosed with dementia an average of 23 years later.
- Of patients with dementia, 1,136 were diagnosed with Alzheimer's disease and 416 with vascular dementia.

Researchers say that people who smoked more than two packs of cigarettes a day in middle age had an elevated risk of dementia overall and also of each subtype, Alzheimer's and vascular dementia, compared with nonsmokers.

Slideshow: 13 Best Quit-Smoking Tips Ever
Former Smokers

On the other hand, former smokers or people who smoked less than half a pack per day did not appear to be at increased risk of developing dementia. And associations between dementia and smoking did not vary by race or sex.

Smoking is considered a well-established risk factor for stroke and may contribute to the risk of vascular dementia through similar mechanisms, the researchers say.

In addition, they say that smoking contributes to oxidative stress and inflammation, which are believed to be important in the development of Alzheimer's disease.

"It is possible that smoking affects the development of dementia via vascular and neurodegenerative pathways," the researchers write.

Previously, a link between smoking and the risk of Alzheimer's disease has been considered controversial, with some studies even suggesting that smoking reduces the risk of cognitive impairment, Parkinson's disease, and other neurodegenerative conditions.

Although smoking's ill effect on public health has been well established, the researcher say, this study shows its impact is likely to become even greater as the population ages and dementia prevalence increases.

The study shows heavy smoking was found to be associated with a greater than 100% increase in risk of dementia and its forms 20 years after midlife, and that the brain is thus "not immune to long-term consequences of heavy smoking."

Appendix E: Do Aricept and Namenda really help Alzheimer's symptoms?

An anonymous caregiver asked...
My mother has Alzheimer's and we are considering taking her off of her medications of Namenda and Aricept. She was diagnosed 12 years ago and is in the late moderate to early severe stage, probably between 6 and 7. I am not convinced this medication is helping, not to mention it's VERY expensive. She takes many many medications and the costs are getting very difficult for her to pay. I'm looking to see what experience others may have with family members taking these two drugs and if they believe it helps. I think it possibly helped for awhile but she is declining fairly quickly now and I'm no so sure it's helping any longer. Thanks

Terrysmith700 said...

I agree that these medicines are not helpful in the late stages. The owner of the last facility where my mother resided, before coming to my home, always said she had never seen them help anyone in her 20 years of offering the service. I think you have to be very careful about discontinuing these meds...they start off introducing them slowly into the patients system so stopping abruptly could present problems. You should check with her doctor before taking action. In my mothers case the assisted living facility that she was in failed to provide the proper dosage (I monitored the Rx refills on my mother's medicines and could tell from the frequency of the refill and the amount left in the bottle after a 30 day period). So I knew that she was getting less over a period of time so the prescribed frequency was easy to reduce after that. However, I did notice some increased agitation, but could not tie it to her reduced intake of Namenda. These meds are expensive and I think they are not helpful for memory issues. Bless you in your effort, I know how hard this is.

D.A.H. said...

Our Mom is in the middle stages of Alzheimer's, and she was on Aricept for about 2 weeks. She was so ill, that we took her off of it. She lives alone, and the side effects of this drug were so awful (vomiting, increased confusion, dizziness and headaches) that we worried about her even more. Maybe she was just more sensitive than other people, but it just wasn't worth it. Besides, there's no guarantee that the symptoms would abate...there was no sign that there we lessening with our Mom, and she was completely miserable. Now she's happier, side effects gone. The decision to take her off Aricept may not have been the best decision, but her quality of life (however much more time she has), is of utmost importance to us.

ctconnie said...

My Dad was on both Aricept and Namenda for 2-3 years; the Aricept was just stopped and he's still getting Namenda. I think they helped the disease slow down, but how does anyone really know?? His Aricept was stopped once by his primary care doc, who didn't think he needed it. He immediately had lots more confusion, so we restarted it. Now he's advanced in the disease, and the nursing home staff are worried about his declining appetite, which is why they stopped it this time. They started him on Risperdal instead. He is doing OK.

I don't really understand why he's still on Namenda.

I HATE THIS AWFUL DISEASE!!!!!

CLC said...

Like your situation, my Dad is now showing Stage 7 signs (some difficulty swallowing solids). He's on Namenda and Aricept as well (didn't tolerate Exelon at all, vomiting etc.). I have read that in later stages AD Namenda and Aricept are no longer effective in delaying the effects of the disease - so taking them much longer seems pointless. As long as he recognizes us, and can function well in terms of eating, bathing, dressing and socializing, we will continue them, and stop when the situation turns. However, I can tell you I shudder to think how much faster he would have progressed without them. He's had nine high functioning years since diagnosis, which he might not have had without them. I have no idea how families without means handle the cost - at least he has a decent enough pension to get by.

But our family has an additional wrinkle: he also takes a dozen or so medications for heart, high blood pressure and so on. My brother and I (along with his cardiologist, whose mother also died of AD) also feel that force feeding pills for heart disease to ward off a heart attack or related is also pointless, given his stage of AD. None of the pills can cure his cardio issues. All they do is allow him to live long enough to ultimately die of AD. He has signed advanced directives, and under that auspice, we are considering weaning him in the next few months from his cardiac meds as well. We would rather he pass relatively quickly -and naturally - from cardio failure, than struggle (with us) through end stage AD. He always said he'd rather die with a hammer in his hand than be hooked up with tubes, so we are taking his philosophy to heart.

Has anyone else faced this dilemma of two competing and ultimately terminal diseases?

A fellow caregiver said...

My mother is in the middle stages of Alzheimer's. She tried Aricept but it made her extremely nauseous so we stopped it after 2 weeks.

However later she started having more episodes of being nervous - so the Dr. tried her on Namenda which has been very effective on calming her, with no apparent side effects.

CLC said...

CTConnie: you should check out Risperdal as it has a track record of sudden and fatal heart attacks in dementia patients. It's primarily used for schizophrenia and bipolar conditions, but can promote weight gain, which may be why they prescribed it. Just beware of the potential risks, even though he seems to be doing better. One listing from many returns on a search: http://www.rxlist.com/risperdal-drug.htm.

ctconnie said...

CLC - thanks, yes, I checked it out prior to giving them the OK to start it. I am aware of the risks. His quality of life is so poor, a sudden heart attack would be a welcome end to all of our suffering.

A fellow caregiver said...

Don't know if this is an answer exactly but -- please share the following article: http://www.huffingtonpost.com/2009/06/12/eli-lillys-zyprexa-fraud_n_214907.html, or google: Eli Lillys Zyprexa fraud. This past week, news stories from several sources have come forth that Eli Lilly and 2 other leading drug companies have been caught lying about the qualities attributed to Zyprexa and other drugs. The drugs are not what the drug companies said they were and even though research labs denied what the drug companies said, these major pharmaceuticals were still allowed to market their drugs erroneously. Lilly and Pfizer have both been fined, but not forced to stop marketing these drugs. It's not just Alzheimer's drugs I know, but if people do not know what's going on, drug companies will continue to sell expensive, ineffective and even dangerous drugs. Before you allow your loved ones to take drugs, google or research them first.

Hi,

My mother's doctor has indicated that none of these drugs really work in late stages, and he questioned whether they did much of anything in earlier stages. My mother's prior doctor put her on Aricept and then added the Namenda, mainly because the drug company was pushing it and I don't think he really had a clue about my mother's condition. Current doctor said to take her off Namenda and ensure she has 10mg of Aricept at her current stage, but that both drugs together were unnecessary at this stage and expensive. I would really question the doctor about the scripts. Also, my mother seems to have a good deal of nausea, which I think is related to the medication. It makes her feel physically worse so it is on my agenda to discuss with her doctor at her next appt. If he thinks we can take her off all of it, I intend to give it a shot. However, getting him to do that and getting her to go along with it are two different things! I can't seem to get my mother to quit having the pharmacy refill both Rx's even though her doctor told her two months ago to only take the Aricept! At this point, I'm about ready to start taking them myself to see if it will help ME!!! Starting to feel like I am the one with the problem.

An anonymous caregiver said...

I agree that the drugs are effective in the early stages of AD, but are much less so in the later stages. My mother was taking both Aricept and Namenda. She tolerated them well and her dementia spanned about a 5 year period. She was able to live at home (with help) until she died suddenly of a stroke at home. Right before she died I was considering discontinuing the medications because her quality of life was diminishing rapidly. She would have been mortified had she been able to realize the degree of her confusion and dependence on others. It was a true blessing and my hope that my mother would die suddenly and at home, because I had seen first hand that being hospitalized is very confusing for patients with dementia and most of them experience extreme anxiety and disorientation. I feel the drugs are good in the beginning of the disease, but once the quality of life goes down they do little good, except to prolong the sad journey. I feel that to remove excessive medications, including those for heart disease can be a blessing because a sudden death is so much kinder for elderly people. My mother died in her own kitchen over a 10 to 15 minute period after collapsing and becoming unconscious. It was traumatic at the time, especially for my father, who was at her side. However, when I arrived at the scene 10 or 15 minutes later and found her sitting peacefully and lifeless in her own chair at the table, I knew she had died in a way she would have chosen for herself and with dignity. I cannot begin to describe the aura of peace that surrounded her. It is important to remember that doctors are forced to practice "defensive medicine" to avoid lawsuits. They usually offer all options and often patients are taking medicines or undergoing "state-of-the-art" treatments that really aren't helping. I say this without bitterness because I am a doctor. It becomes the family's responsibility to access the effectiveness and practicality of treatment. If your loved one makes his/her wishes known before losing the capacity to care for himself/herself, it is much easier to allow nature to take its course without feeling guilty. It is always a hard choice. I would urge anyone who has a parent with early stage dementia to discuss their end of life wishes. If you know that your parent does not want to be hooked to life support, given IV nutrition or fluids, or take life-prolonging medication when there is no hope for cure it is much easier to carry out their wishes without feeling the guilt of making life and death decisions for another person.

My mother has been on Namenda for about 3 years and it was prescribed to diminish the hallucinations due to her Dementia, which is still currently mild to mid. This med has helped with the hallucinations significantly over other meds, including Aricept, which gave her nausea. We tried several other meds before settling on Namenda, and this has been the best so far, no side effects, and I'm grateful for it now, though I know the disease will continue to deteriorate. Alzheimer's/Dementia is so prevalent now it makes me wonder if in times past there was so much of this disease-are we a now product of of our culture and environment? We try to band-aid this disease with all sorts of costly pills and meds, but are there efforts to try to find the root of all of this- for our generation? I realize we have to deal with the current problem now, but I hope for the future of our kids who will caregive us, that there are efforts being made now to get to the bottom of it!

My answer is directed to the doctor who suggested stopping heart meds.......I shudder to think that people will read your comment and consider an end of life choice NOT to prolong death by false means will include medications prescribed and taken for many years at their own choice. Doctor, you are tipping on the edge of the G O D syndrome...there are some very stressed and unstable care providers reading and writing in this venue and you are implying to stop the meds that preserve life in their loved ones...I am shocked and disturbed.

An anonymous caregiver said...

It is fascinating that there are so many different answers to a question. We are also saying "doctor said" which makes me ask what credentials they hold. Are they neurologists or specialists? My husband has been on Aricept and then Namenda for about 6 years. He is in his 9th year of Alzheimer's and Lewy body dementia. He is now in hospice care. I feel that we have had all of these great years because of these two medicines which were started early. I also have asked his neurologist if they should be discontinued and her answer was, No, because we can't be sure what help they are still giving at this point. He is also on medicine for heart conditions. Last week he had a minor stroke and is beginning his transition. He is at peace, comfortable, and very content. He can still move, talk, sit in a wheelchair, and go to the dining room to eat some. We can still talk and he understands me and indicates that with his eye movements. Do I discontinue any meds when the man is so comfortable and content? I am glad that I have more than one doctor and hospice to give me guidance.

pollytnjc said...

Hi,

You are so right that it makes a difference the credentials of the doctor. In my mother's case, she would only see an internist who just kept throwing any drug at her without even assessing where she was. NOW she is seeing a neurologist who specializes in Alzheimer's and he is taking a more cautious approach. He is thinking she is not ready for Namenda, and wants her dosage on Aricept at 10mg as she is early/borderline mid-stage Alzheimer's. I think the problem, even with specialists, is that this disease progresses differently for everyone, drugs or no drugs, and the jury is still out on whether any of them truly help. Your husband may be someone who would have gone more slowly anyway, or the drug may have really worked for him. Frankly, I feel we are all in one big experiment. I think you are right to continue the drugs - they are obviously not hurting him, and I wouldn't mess with anything right now if I were you. You sound like you are getting the best help available for your husband. He is fortunate to have you. I am so glad for you that you can still enjoy each other's company. I love my mother and cherish our time together. It is still very hard, however, and some days I believe that the two of us would benefit most if I were on the drugs! In any case, best wishes to you both.

An anonymous caregiver said...

Terrysmith700: And how does shoving medications into an individual to "preserve life" also not play into the God-syndrome? If one were true to the "let it be" or "god's will" mentality, one would withhold all medications and let nature take it's course. I cannot for the life of me, understand the rationale of pre-lifers who would condemn both patient and family to the anguish of a prolonged and grisly death thru end stage AD, when simply weaning an AD patient with chronic and severe cardiac issues of their meds would simply allow nature to determine whether heart or neuro ends life. If anything screams "I will keep you alive whether you want it or not", shoving meds that offer no cure into a terminal patient, that is it. The medicator is in control, not nature, not a Divine authority. Please, stop the "suffering is part of dying" nonsense and associated guilt trips and let families and their physicians who know the patient determine a course of final treatment, such as it may be.

CLC said...

Terrysmith700: And what if the patient has an advanced directive? At what point do medications that frankly offer very little other than another day of misery and pain become an artificial intervention of modern science? If I were to read between the lines, my bet is you, as a family member would fight a DNR or advanced directive to stop treatments that offered no hope of cure. What is the difference between decreasing or discontinuing redundant cardiac meds on a terminal AD patient (and they are) and shutting off life support on a brain dead patient? Or would you just keep the ventilator going ad infinitum? I fully understand that many caregivers are at the end of their ropes, and your have legitimate concerns about the potential for desparate actions. I don't think the original author was making this a call to action - in fact, I think the author was looking for input if you reread the original post.

It is a tough call, a call made (hopefully) with full appreciation of the wishes of the patient. I think that many (certainly not all) doctors recognize that there is a huge ethical conflict and personal angst in proscribing treatments that prolong 'technical' life in the face of imminent death or prolonged life support with no hope of recovery. We have become victims of medicine and technology advances; there is a great deal of appeal to the time when shamans treated the dying with pain medicines while the family waited and prayed to their Divine Spirit to take their loved one quickly and painlessly to the other side. If anyone is now playing 'God', it's the health care service that 'preserves life' in direct conflict with the admonition to "do no harm."

And yes, for the record, I personally believe with proper oversight by non-bureaucrats, psychologists and spiritual advisors that end of life assistance to terminally ill patients should be legalized. Disagree as you will, but a competent patient should have such a right. Your soul made the decision to come into this life; it ought to have the option to exit.

confused said...

My mom took Namenda, for about 1year it was not helping here at all so the family weaned her off of it and went back to what she was taking for her mood swings and also her wandering. The med she was taking and still taking is called Mirtazapine that has been treating her well. Her mood swings are down and has slowed down with the wandering.

I agree with you 100%. My Mom has a Living Will/Advanced Directives that we are following. I am very sorry for your loss.

On another note. Namenda helps dementia patients follow commands but really doesn't work in the end stages.

pallcaredoc said...

This a tough one. My sense from patients I've seen over the years is the later stage of the disease, the less useful these drugs are and therefore the greater relative burden of cost and side effects. I would be interested in hearing the experiences of caregivers who have stopped these drugs in late stage disease. Was there a noticeable difference? Any change in appetite, social functioning, or ability to care for oneself?

With regard to the cardiac meds I would make sure you understand what the medicine is for. If its to prolong life, certainly it is reasonable to stop it since prolonging life is no longer an appropriate goal. But if it is to prevent chest pain, shortness of breath, or rapid heart rate leading to dizziness and falls, it may be best to continue it.

Finally, regarding psychotropics (antipsychotics) they should be used only for intractable agitation and hallucinations, and continued only if they are clearly helping. I explain the risk of sudden death to family members, but frankly this may not be a great concern when the patient is suffering terribly.

joyg said...

My husband had been on both of these drugs since 2001. When his last year was spent under hospice care, we discussed this quite a bit. The conclusion was that he should stay on them. You never know how they are still working for the patient and that therefore it is much better to keep them going. This from the hospice team who is quite qualified and trying to just keep the patient comfortable.

Jan99 said...
My mother has been on Namenda & Exelon for over 3.5 years now, Exelon about 5. Namenda helped her tremendously. It halted her dementia decline, with no noticeable decline at all. In fact, she improved. It could be a combination of Namenda, living at home under my care, removing her from the awful nursing home w/ uncaring staffs, exercises, stimulating activities at her Adult Day Health Care (for Alzheimer's), and other changes. She is doing amazingly well at 99. She has no other medical problems except for dementia, high BP & atrial fibrillation.

Appendix F: Voyager Pharmaceuticals Press Release

For Immediate Release
Novel Approach May Offer New Hope to Women with Alzheimer's Disease, Study Shows
Drug that lowers pituitary hormone maintains functional capabilities for a longer period of time Madrid, Spain (July 17, 2006) – Leuprolide acetate helps women with mild-to-moderate Alzheimer's disease maintain functional capabilities for a longer period of time, according to data presented Monday by **Voyager Pharmaceutical Corporation.** The company shared its findings from a Phase II clinical trial in women at a symposium held during the 10th International Conference on Alzheimer's Disease and Related Disorders, presented by the Alzheimer's Association. This report expanded on the Phase II data presented in Geneva, Switzerland in April by Dr. Brian Reynolds, director of medical and scientific information for **Voyager.** "Women treated with leuprolide acetate and the current standard of care, acetylcholinesterase inhibitors, better maintained their level of cognitive ability and daily activities for nearly one year," said Dr. Christopher Gregory, vice president of research at Voyager.

"These findings mean that, for a sustained period of time, women treated with the drug were able to maintain their memory and their ability to do like things like dress themselves."

The findings resulted from a subgroup analysis of VP-AD-103, Voyager's clinical trial testing the efficacy and safety of leuprolide acetate in women with mild-to-moderate Alzheimer's disease. The trial was a 48-week, double-blind, placebo-controlled study observing women age 65 and older. The subgroup analysis compared two groups of women with mild-to-moderate Alzheimer's disease. The first group consisted of women treated with leuprolide acetate and acetylcholinesterase inhibitors (AChEIs). The second group consisted of women treated with placebo and AChEIs. Women in the study were assessed on three measures: cognitive ability (measured by an assessment known as ADAS-Cog), clinical impression (a physician and caregiver assessment known as ADCS-CGIC), and ability to perform daily activities (as assessed by the caregiver on a scale known as ADCS-ADL). The treatment group performed significantly better than the placebo group on all three measures. Nearly 90 percent of the eligible women from the Phase II trial elected to participate in an open-label extension study. Results from that study showed that women continued to benefit from treatment with leuprolide acetate for
nearly one more year. "Our trial result demonstrates that leuprolide acetate may benefit a spectrum of women with mild to-moderate Alzheimer's disease for a sustained period of time," said Dr. Joseph DeVeaugh-Geiss, Voyager's interim chief medical officer. "These findings are encouraging as we continue to make progress with our trials in Alzheimer's disease." Voyager is currently enrolling subjects for two Phase III clinical trials investigating the safety and efficacy of VP4896 (leuprolide

acetate implant) in the treatment of mild-to-moderate Alzheimer's disease. Enrollment for the first trial is well ahead of schedule. Voyager expects to complete enrollment of all 555 subjects before Dec. 31, 2006. At ICAD 2006, members of Voyager's team will also be presenting four scientific/clinical posters relating to the Phase I and II clinical trials, preclinical research linking leuprolide acetate to AD pathology and a "Hot Topics" poster that addresses data from both of Voyager's Phase II studies.

About the Phase II Study: The data presented are the results of a subgroup analysis of Voyager's 48-week double blind, placebo-controlled Phase II study. The study assessed the efficacy and safety of leuprolide acetate in stabilizing cognitive and global function in women age 65 and older with mild-to moderate Alzheimer's disease. The primary efficacy endpoints of the trial were scores on both the ADAS-Cog (a test of memory and cognition) and the ADCS-CGIC (a global measure of a subject's change in condition) at 48 weeks compared to baseline.

There were various secondary efficacy endpoints, including scores on the ADCS-ADL (a measurement of a patient's capacity to perform activities of daily living) at 48 weeks compared to baseline. In the subgroup analysis, the mean ADAS-Cog score in the group receiving the high dose of leuprolide acetate and an AChEI declined by 0.18 points from baseline at week 48 compared to a mean decline of 3.30 points in the group receiving placebo and an AChEI. In the ADCS-CGIC analysis, 58 percent of the subgroup receiving the high dose of leuprolide acetate and an AChEI scored no change or better at week 48 in comparison with baseline versus 38 percent of the subgroup receiving placebo and an AChEI. The mean ADCS-ADL score in the subgroup receiving the high dose of leuprolide acetate and an AChEI declined 0.54 points from baseline at week 48 compared to a mean decline of 6.85 points in the subgroup receiving placebo and an AChEI. About Voyager Pharmaceutical Corporation Voyager Pharmaceutical Corporation is a biopharmaceutical company focused on developing drugs for diseases associated with aging and development. Voyager's scientific approach is based on the observation that many diseases of aging may be caused by changes in human reproductive hormone levels that are characteristic of the aging process. Voyager's most advanced product candidate is VP4896, a proprietary, small, biodegradable implant that is comprised of leuprolide acetate and a polymer. VP4896 decreases the amount of luteinizing hormone (LH) released by the pituitary gland.

Based on clinical evidence, Voyager believes that the reduction of LH may decrease or slow the progression of Alzheimer's disease. The active ingredient in VP4896, leuprolide acetate, has been used safely for over 20 years as a treatment for prostate cancer. Voyager's phase III trial program for VP4896 is investigating the effects of this new AD therapy on the rate of cognitive decline in mild-to-moderate Alzheimer's disease.

Voyager was founded in 2001 and is headquartered in Raleigh, N.C. For more information go to www.voyagerpharma.com

Overview of Voyager Pharmaceuticals

We are a biopharmaceutical company focused on developing drugs for diseases associated with aging and development. Our most advanced product candidate is **Memryte**, a proprietary, small, biodegradable implant that is comprised of leuprolide acetate and a polymer, that we are developing for the treatment of mild to moderate Alzheimer's disease. Leuprolide acetate has been widely used over the past 20 years for the treatment of a number of hormone-related disorders, such as prostate cancer, endometriosis and precocious puberty, and has a well-established safety record in humans.

In the third quarter of 2005, we initiated enrollment and dosed the first patient in the first of our two randomized, double blind, placebo controlled, 56-week, pivotal Phase III clinical trials of the Memryte implant for the treatment of mild to moderate Alzheimer's disease as adjunctive therapy with acetylcholinesterase inhibitors, or ACIs. We plan to initiate enrollment in the second Phase III clinical trial in the fourth quarter of 2005. We expect to enroll approximately 550 patients in each of these trials. ACIs are the most widely prescribed current therapy for Alzheimer's disease and include Aricept, Reminyl, also known as Razadyne, Exelon and Cognex. We reviewed the study protocol and statistical analyses for these two pivotal Phase III clinical trials with the Division of Neuropharmacological Drug Products of the Center for Drug Evaluation and Research of the FDA in August 2005. The FDA agreed to our clinical development plan and indicated that the results from our clinical trials to date were adequate for us to initiate our Phase III trials.

Alzheimer's disease is a progressive, degenerative and ultimately terminal brain disorder that gradually destroys a person's memory and ability to learn, reason, make judgments, communicate and carry out daily activities. There is currently no treatment that stops or materially slows the progression of Alzheimer's disease. As a result, it is one of the world's largest unmet medical needs. Direct and indirect annual costs of caring for individuals with Alzheimer's disease in the United States are at least $100 billion, according to estimates used by the Alzheimer's Association and the National Institute on Aging. The global market for currently available Alzheimer's disease drugs is growing rapidly and was over $3 billion in 2004. The American Health Assistance Foundation estimates that approximately 18 million people worldwide, including approximately 4.5 million people in the United States, suffer from Alzheimer's disease.

We recently completed a randomized, double blind, placebo controlled, 48-week, Phase II dose-ranging clinical trial of an injectable formulation of leuprolide acetate in 108 women aged 65 or older as a treatment for mild to moderate Alzheimer's disease. Although Phase II clinical results may not be predictive of results in subsequent clinical trials, in this Phase II trial, there was a trend at week 48 in favor of the high dose leuprolide acetate group indicating a relative stabilization of the disease compared to the placebo group. In addition, in a prospective subgroup analysis of patients who were taking ACIs, the group of 24 patients who also received the high dose of leuprolide acetate demonstrated a benefit over the group of 26 patients who were treated with placebo. In our pivotal Phase III trials, the primary efficacy endpoints involve studying the efficacy of the Memryte implant as adjunctive therapy with ACIs. Accordingly, we do not expect to perform subgroup analyses.

In addition to our recently completed Phase II clinical trial of leuprolide acetate in women, we have completed enrollment and are conducting a similar randomized, double blind, placebo controlled, 48-week, Phase II dose-ranging clinical trial of an injectable formulation of leuprolide acetate in 119 men, which we expect to complete in the second quarter of 2006. Although not statistically significant, interim analysis of the data from the 33 patients enrolled in the trial who had reached week 26 at the time of the analysis showed a trend in favor of the groups receiving leuprolide acetate in comparison with the group receiving placebo. The results of this interim analysis were derived from a small number of patients and were not designed to demonstrate statistical significance.

Appendix G: Voyager Pharmaceuticals' Therapeutic Approach to Alzheimer's

Alzheimer's disease is named after Dr. Alois Alzheimer, a German physician, who first described the disease in 1906. Alzheimer's disease is a progressive, degenerative and ultimately terminal brain disorder that gradually destroys a person's memory and ability to learn, reason, make judgments, communicate and carry out daily activities. Alzheimer's disease patients may also experience changes in personality and behavior, such as anxiety, suspiciousness and agitation, as well as delusions or hallucinations as the disease progresses. Alzheimer's disease is invariably associated with, and defined by, the loss of connections between, and the death of, neurons, as well as deposits of beta amyloid plaque and the formation of neurofibrillary tangles in the brain. Existing approved therapies treat the symptoms of some patients with Alzheimer's disease by temporarily enhancing a patient's cognitive function and general behavior for a period of time; however, there is no existing treatment that stops or materially slows Alzheimer's disease progression. Unless the patient first succumbs to some other disease, Alzheimer's disease eventually leads to the patient's total incapacitation and ultimately to death.

Alzheimer's disease is an age-related disease. The Alzheimer's Association estimates that 10% of all individuals over the age of 65 suffer from Alzheimer's disease and that nearly 50% of all individuals who reach age 85 suffer from Alzheimer's disease. The Alzheimer's Health Assistance Foundation estimates that approximately 350,000 new cases of Alzheimer's disease are diagnosed annually in the United States. Alzheimer's disease is roughly twice as prevalent in women as in men. Alzheimer's disease onset has been reported in Down's

Syndrome individuals aged as young as 30, with a dramatic increase in prevalence with aging. Approximately 18 million people worldwide suffer from Alzheimer's disease, including an estimated 4.5 million Americans, more than double the number of Americans suffering from this disease in 1980.

The Alzheimer's Association reports that Alzheimer's disease patients live an average of eight years, with many patients living as much as 20 years, from the initial onset of symptoms. Direct and indirect annual costs of caring for individuals with Alzheimer's disease in the United States are at least $100 billion, according to estimates used by the Alzheimer's Association and the National Institute on Aging. The Alzheimer's Association estimates the average lifetime cost of care for an individual with Alzheimer's disease in the United States to be approximately $174,000.

Historically, Alzheimer's disease has been diagnosed through testing of the patient using measures of memory, thinking skills and the capacity to perform activities of daily living. There is ongoing research in the field of neuroimaging, including the use of magnetic resonance imaging, or MRIs, and positron emission tomography, or PET, scans to assist in the diagnosis of Alzheimer's disease. Some researchers believe that these brain imaging techniques may permit identification of changes in brain appearance or function in advance of the development of cognitive or behavioral symptoms of Alzheimer's disease. If Alzheimer's disease can be diagnosed presymptomatically, it may be possible to treat patients earlier in the disease process and for longer periods *of time.*

Beta Amyloid Hypothesis of Alzheimer's Disease

There are several hypotheses regarding the cause of Alzheimer's disease, the predominant one being the beta amyloid hypothesis. The assumption behind this hypothesis is that amyloid beta protein, which makes up the plaques present in the brains of Alzheimer's disease patients, is toxic and is the causative agent of the disease. The generally accepted view is that inhibiting the production of, and enhancing the clearance of, amyloid beta protein plaques may prevent or treat Alzheimer's disease. Based on this hypothesis, many companies have designed therapies to suppress or eliminate amyloid beta protein in order to affect the rate of progression of Alzheimer's disease. Research based on the beta amyloid hypothesis has been ongoing for two decades without yielding any approved therapies to date.

Cell Cycle Hypothesis of Alzheimer's Disease

The cell cycle hypothesis of Alzheimer's disease, which is relatively new and has not achieved the same wide acceptance as the beta amyloid hypothesis, proposes that all of the known neurological and biochemical changes associated with Alzheimer's disease are caused by the abnormal re-entry of brain cells into the cell division cycle, or process by which one cell replicates itself and divides into two cells. In general, it is thought that adult brain cells do not divide. Thus, this hypothesis suggests that when adult brain cells are stimulated to divide, the neurological changes seen in Alzheimer's disease result. The proponents of this hypothesis believe that the cell cycle process in Alzheimer's disease is triggered by the presence of an unknown mitogen, or substance that stimulates this cell division.

A number of recent studies and scientific publications provide support for the validity of the cell cycle hypothesis. For example, a study published in *The Journal of Neuroscience* in April 1998 (Jonathan Busser, David S. Geldmacher and Karl Herrup: *Ectopic Cell Cycle Proteins Predict the Sites of Neuronal Cell Death in Alzheimer's Disease Brain*, 18(8): 2801-2807) comparing the brain tissue from autopsy specimens of Alzheimer's disease patients with that of persons without Alzheimer's disease proposed that various components of the cell cycle contribute significantly to regionally specific neuronal death in Alzheimer's disease. More recently, in 2003, a review published in *Progress in Cell Cycle Research* (Inez Vincent, Chong In Pae and Janice L. Hallows: *The cell cycle and human neurodegenerative disease*, Vol. 5: 31-41 (2003)) referred to accumulating evidence suggesting that aberrant activation of the cell cycle in some neurodegenerative diseases leads to the death of neurons. The review also noted that the apparent involvement of cell cycle dysregulation in neurodegeneration creates therapeutic potential to curb the onset and progression of degenerative diseases. Also in 2003, a review published in *Progress in Neurobiology* (Thomas Arendt: *Synaptic plasticity and cell cycle activation in neurons are alternative effector pathways: the 'Dr. Jekyll and Mr. Hyde concept' of Alzheimer's disease or the yin and yang of neuroplasticity,* 71 (2003): 83-248) asserted that preventing cell cycle activation will be crucial to preventing neurodegeneration, or nerve cell death. Our research efforts to date and our development of Memryte have been based in part on such publications and our belief that LH is the mitogen that drives brain cells into abnormal cell division, thereby causing Alzheimer's disease.

Human Reproductive Hormone Feedback Loop

The concentration of certain hormones secreted by the hypothalamus area of the brain, the pituitary gland and the gonads is regulated by a feedback loop. The loop is initiated by proteins called activins that stimulate the hypothalamus to release gonadotropin-releasing hormone, or GnRH. GnRH then stimulates the pituitary to secrete the two gonadotropins—LH and follicle-stimulating hormone, or FSH. The gonadotropins bind to receptors on the gonads, the ovaries in females and the testicles in males, and stimulate and regulate the production of eggs in females and sperm in males. The gonadotropins also stimulate the gonads to produce the sex steroid hormones, estrogen and testosterone.

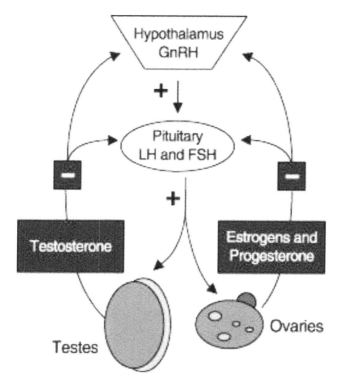

Once the hypothalamus senses that the sex steroid hormones are at an acceptable level, it reduces the release of GnRH. The reduced level of GnRH provides feedback to the pituitary gland to reduce the secretion of gonadotropins, resulting in reduced gonadotropin levels. Reduced gonadotropin levels then provide feedback to the gonads to reduce the production of the sex steroid hormones. Once the hypothalamus senses the sex steroid hormones dropping below a particular level, the hypothalamus increases the release of GnRH, which re-initiates the hormonal feedback loop and the production of the two gonadotropins.

Our Scientific Approach

Our scientific approach is based on the observation that many diseases of aging may be caused by the age-related changes in levels of reproductive hormones that are secreted by the hypothalamus area of the brain, the pituitary gland and the gonads. This approach is built on the premise that these hormones are beneficial early in life, because they regulate and promote development and growth through cell division and differentiation in order to achieve reproduction, but are harmful later in life because, in an attempt to maintain reproduction and fertility, they become unregulated and cause abnormal cell division. We believe that this change in hormone levels is a primary cause of many age-related diseases, including Alzheimer's disease, various cancers and Parkinson's disease.

We believe that the gonadotropin LH is the mitogen that causes Alzheimer's disease. Our research suggests that LH serves as the catalyst that causes brain cells to abnormally divide and that LH potentially leads to increased production of amyloid beta protein. We base these beliefs on both experimental evidence and scientific observations, principally resulting from our work and the work of our consultants, including:

- In a study published in the *Journal of Neuroendocrinology* in April 2000, which was authored by Richard L. Bowen, our Chief Scientific Officer (R. L. Bowen: *An Association of Elevated Serum Gonadotropin Concentrations and Alzheimer's Disease?*, Vol. 12: 351-354) regarding the analysis of circulating levels of LH in the blood of 40 patients diagnosed with Alzheimer's disease compared to 29 age-matched patients with no Alzheimer's disease diagnosis, the average concentration of LH in the blood of the Alzheimer's disease patients was significantly higher than the average concentration of LH in the blood of patients with no Alzheimer's disease diagnosis;

- In a study published in the *Journal of Neuroscience Research* in 2002, which was co-authored by Richard L. Bowen, our Chief Scientific Officer (Richard L. Bowen, Mark A. Smith, Peggy L.R. Harris, Zvezdana Kybat, Ralph N. Martins, Rudolph J. Castellani, George Perry and Craig T. Atwood, 70: 514-518) regarding the analysis of human brain tissue from autopsy specimens, LH levels in brains of cases diagnosed with Alzheimer's disease were found to be twice as high as in brains of cases without Alzheimer's disease, with the highest concentrations of LH found in the parts of the brain known to be vulnerable to Alzheimer's disease related damage;

- In cell culture tests, LH stimulated an increase in the rate of division of human brain cancer cells and resulted in the death of normal adult mouse brain cells;

- In cell culture tests, human brain cancer cells treated with LH showed a two-fold increase in amyloid beta protein production over untreated cells;

- In a study published in *The Journal of Biological Chemistry* in 2004, which was co-authored by Richard L. Bowen, our Chief Scientific Officer (Richard L. Bowen, Guiseppe Verdile, Tianbing Liu, Albert F. Parlow, George Perry, Mark A. Smith, Ralph N. Martins and Craig S. Atwood: *Luteinizing Hormone, a Reproductive Regulator That Modulates the Processing of Amyloid-ß Precursor Protein and Amyloid-ß Deposition*, Vol., 279, No. 19, Issue of May 7: 20539-20545) in a mouse model of Alzheimer's disease, animals treated with leuprolide acetate exhibited 50% less amyloid beta protein than animals treated with placebo; and

- In a mouse model of Alzheimer's disease, animals treated with leuprolide acetate demonstrated an ability to preserve memory function while the mice treated with placebo did not.

We also base our belief that LH is the mitogen causing Alzheimer's disease on other evidence, much of which is based on the well-established observation that there are many similarities between the Alzheimer's disease brain and the fetal brain, including:

- LH is very similar to human chorionic gonadotropin,

or hCG, the hormone detected by urine pregnancy tests, and is known to work through the same receptor. hCG is elevated during fetal development and may be important for brain growth, a process associated with rapid brain cell division;

• In both the Alzheimer's disease brain and the fetal brain, the cell division cycle is highly activated;

• In both the Alzheimer's disease brain and the fetal brain, very high levels of hyperphosphorylated tau protein, which makes up the neurofibrillary tangles found in Alzheimer's disease, are present;

• In both the Alzheimer's disease brain and the fetal brain, there is increased processing of amyloid precursor protein, which is used to make the amyloid found in the plaques of the Alzheimer's disease brain; and

• In both the Alzheimer's disease brain and the fetal brain, there is an increase in presenelin-1, an enzyme associated with amyloid processing.

Finally, individuals with Down's Syndrome have elevated levels of gonadotropin throughout their lives and often develop Alzheimer's disease-like pathology in their 30's. Males with Down's syndrome have much higher levels of gonadotropin and develop Alzheimer's disease-like pathology earlier in life than their female counterparts, the reversal of the pattern for Alzheimer's disease observed in the general population.

If the gonadotropin LH is the mitogen that causes abnormal cell division in the brain or if LH leads to the production of amyloid beta protein and either of these factors causes Alzheimer's disease, we believe it may be possible to prevent or treat Alzheimer's disease by controlling a person's LH levels. We are seeking to do this with leuprolide acetate, which is a GnRH analog that, when administered to a human being, causes an initial increase in LH and FSH levels, followed by a precipitous and sustained decline in the levels of these hormones. This decrease occurs as a result of the down regulation and desensitization of pituitary GnRH receptors. At physiologic dosage levels, leuprolide acetate is effective at suppressing LH to a level that is undetectable in the bloodstream.

Limitations of Current Alzheimer's Disease Therapies

There are currently five drugs approved for the treatment of Alzheimer's disease in the United States:

- Aricept, marketed by Pfizer, Inc. and Eisai Company, Ltd.;

- Exelon, marketed by Novartis AG;

- Reminyl, also known as Razadyne, marketed by Shire Pharmaceuticals Group plc and Janssen Pharmaceutical Products, LP;

220

- Cognex, marketed by First Horizon Pharmaceutical Corp; and

- Namenda, marketed by Forest Pharmaceuticals, Inc.

Phase II / ALADDIN I

In December 2004, we completed a randomized, double blind, placebo controlled, dose-ranging, 48-week, Phase II clinical trial to assess the efficacy and safety of an injectable formulation of leuprolide acetate on cognitive and global function in women with mild to moderate Alzheimer's disease. We call this clinical trial ALADDIN I. The trial was conducted at five investigative study sites in the United States. Women aged 65 or older with mild to moderate Alzheimer's disease were eligible to participate in the trial. Patients were allowed to receive ACIs during the trial if they began taking this medication at least 60 days prior to the trial and continued a stable dose throughout the trial.

A total of 109 women were enrolled in this study, 108 of which were included in the intent-to-treat population and assigned to one of three groups comprised of 36 participants each:

- a low dose leuprolide acetate group;

- a high dose leuprolide acetate group; and

- a placebo group.

Each participant was administered an injection of leuprolide acetate or placebo once every 12 weeks during the trial. The primary efficacy endpoints of the trial were a patient's score on the ADAS-Cog and the ADCS-CGIC at 48 weeks compared to baseline. There were various secondary efficacy endpoints, including a patient's score on the ADCS-ADL at 48 weeks compared to baseline. There was a trend at week 48 in favor of the high dose leuprolide acetate group in this Phase II trial indicating a relative stabilization of the disease compared to the placebo group. However, we did not achieve the primary efficacy endpoints or any of the secondary efficacy endpoints in this trial with statistical significance. We believe that the lack of statistical significance was a function in part of the low number of trial participants.

There was also a statistically significant difference in the ADAS-Cog score at 48 weeks in favor of the high dose leuprolide acetate group compared to the low dose leuprolide acetate group. The dose of Memryte being used in our pivotal Phase III clinical trials is based on this result and the interim analysis of our Phase II clinical trial in men.

We also performed a prospective analysis of 78 patients in the intent-to-treat population who were taking ACIs, comparing results for the group of 24 patients treated with ACIs plus the high dose of leuprolide acetate used in the study and the group of 28 patients treated with ACIs plus the low dose of leuprolide acetate used in the study against the results for a group of 26 patients who were treated with ACIs and received placebo in the study. The results for the group that received an ACI plus the low dose of leuprolide acetate were not statistically significantly different from the results for the group that received an ACI plus placebo.

As described below, the group that received the high dose leuprolide acetate plus an ACI demonstrated a benefit in comparison to the group that received an ACI plus placebo. In addition, on each of the seven occasions during the 48-week study at which we assessed these two groups, the mean score of the high dose leuprolide acetate plus ACI group was more favorable than the mean score of the placebo plus ACI group on each of the ADAS-Cog, ADCS-CGIC and ADCS-ADL measures. With respect to ADCS-ADL, which was a secondary efficacy endpoint, the benefit was statistically significant for this subgroup. This subgroup analysis served as the basis of our study design of the Memryte implant as adjunctive therapy with ACIs for our planned pivotal Phase III clinical trials.

Statistical significance is measured by a p-value, which is a mathematical calculation used to determine the statistical meaningfulness of experimental results and indicates the likelihood that the measured result was obtained purely by chance. A p-value of 0.0001 means that the probability that this result occurred by chance is one in 10,000. Statistical significance is usually defined as a p-value of less than 0.05, which means that the probability that this result occurred by chance is less than one in 20. A lower p-value indicates a greater likelihood that the observed result did not occur by chance, and therefore implies greater statistical significance.

For purposes of this subgroup analysis of the results of our ALADDIN I trial, we calculated p-values in two different ways. First we calculated unadjusted p-values, which indicate statistical significance as if this subgroup analysis had been a primary efficacy endpoint. However, because this subgroup analysis was not a primary efficacy endpoint of the ALADDIN I trial, we are required to adjust the p-values for purposes of regulatory determination of statistical significance by applying the Bonferroni correction, which applies an estimated statistical penalty to account for the fact that we have performed an additional analysis of the data. In our pivotal Phase III clinical trials, the primary efficacy endpoints involve studying the efficacy of the Memryte implant as adjunctive therapy with ACIs. Accordingly, we do not expect to perform subgroup analyses and expect that statistical significance will be based only on unadjusted p-values.

In this subgroup analysis, the mean ADAS-Cog score in the group receiving the high dose of leuprolide acetate and an ACI worsened by 0.18 points at week 48 from baseline compared to a mean worsening of 3.30 points in the group receiving placebo and an ACI. The p-value for this difference was 0.026 on an unadjusted basis and 0.078 on an adjusted basis. The following graph illustrates the results of this subgroup analysis of ADAS-Cog scores:

ALADDIN I-Phase II Trial
ADAS-Cog Scores (Intent-to-Treat Analysis)
ACI + High Dose Leuprolide Acetate versus ACI + Placebo

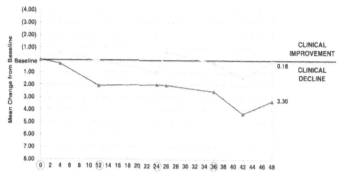

Visit Week (Dosing visit circled; patient assessment dates shown by squares and triangles)

ACI's + High Dose Leuprolide Acetate N [24] —▲— ACI's + Placebo N [26]

In the ADCS-CGIC analysis, 58% of the subgroup receiving the high dose of leuprolide acetate and an ACI scored no change or better at week 48 in comparison with baseline versus 38% of the subgroup receiving placebo and an ACI. The p-value for this difference was 0.031 on an unadjusted basis and 0.093 on an adjusted basis. The following graph illustrates the results of this subgroup analysis of ADCS-CGIC scores:

ALADDIN I-Phase II Trial
ADCS-CGIC Scores (Intent-to-Treat Analysis)
ACI + High Dose Leuprolide Acetate versus ACI + **Placebo**

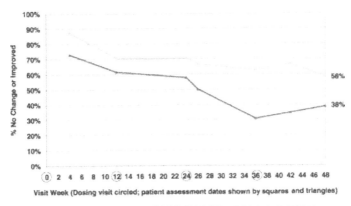

Visit Week (Dosing visit circled; patient assessment dates shown by squares and triangles)

ACI's + High Dose Leuprolide Acetate N [24]   ACI's + Placebo N [26]

The mean ADCS-ADL score in the subgroup receiving the high dose of leuprolide acetate and an ACI declined 0.54 points at week 48 from baseline compared to a mean decline of 6.85 points in the subgroup receiving placebo and an ACI. The p-value for this difference was 0.015 on an unadjusted basis and 0.044 on an adjusted basis.

The following graph illustrates the results of this subgroup analysis of ADCS-ADL scores:

ALADDIN I-Phase II Trial
ADCS-ADL Scores (Intent-to-Treat Analysis)
ACI + High Dose Leuprolide Acetate versus ACI + Placebo

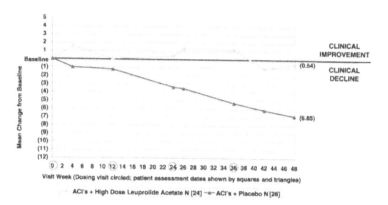

ACI's + High Dose Leuprolide Acetate N [24] — ACI's + Placebo N [26]

The following table summarizes the results of our prospective subgroup analysis of the group that received an ACI plus the high dose of leuprolide acetate versus the group that received an ACI plus placebo in our ALADDIN I trial at 48 weeks:

Summary of ACI Plus High Dose Leuprolide Acetate versus ACI Plus Placebo

Endpoint	ACI + High Dose Leuprolide Acetate (n=24)	ACI + Placebo (n=26)	Unadjusted p-value	Adjusted p-value
ADAS-Cog	0.18point cognitive decline	3.30point cognitive decline	0.026	0.078
ADCS-CGIC	58%no changeor better	38% no change or better	0.031	0.093
ADCS-ADL	0.54point declinein activitiesof daily living	6.85point declinein activitiesof daily living	0.015	0.044

In the ALADDIN I study, leuprolide acetate administered as an injection was well tolerated at both dose levels without any evidence of a dose-related increase in adverse events. Although approximately 77 of the 109 subjects in the ALADDIN I study, or 71%, experienced at least one adverse event, these events were mostly mild or moderate in severity and were mainly regarded as unrelated to the study drug. The most common adverse events reported were consistent with the known safety profile of leuprolide acetate. Twenty serious adverse events were reported in 18 subjects; however, all but three of these adverse events were regarded as not related, or probably not related, and almost certainly were secondary to age, dementia or other underlying disease of the subject. Therefore, no adverse event safety signals of concern were observed in this study. Successful results in completed clinical trials does not mean that subsequent clinical trials will be successful or that such success will be repeated in larger patient populations.

We are currently conducting an open label 96-week extension study to further assess the safety of the high dose of leuprolide acetate, as well as its potential effect on the progression of Alzheimer's disease in patients who completed the 48-week trial. In this extension study, the drug is being administered by injection at 12-week intervals. Of the 73 patients eligible to enroll in the open label extension study, 65 patients, or 89%, elected to do so. We expect to complete this extension study in 2006.

Phase II / ALADDIN II

In December 2003, we initiated a randomized, double blind, placebo controlled, 48-week, Phase II clinical trial designed to assess the efficacy and safety of leuprolide acetate on cognitive and global function in men with Alzheimer's disease. We call this clinical trial ALADDIN II. Men aged 65 or older with mild to moderate Alzheimer's disease are eligible to participate in the trial. The protocol for this trial is substantially similar to the protocol for ALADDIN I. Patients are allowed to receive ACIs during the trial if they began taking this medication at least 60 days prior to the trial and continue a stable dose throughout the trial. We are conducting this Phase II clinical trial at 17 investigative study sites in the United States.

In May 2005, we completed enrollment of a total of 119 trial participants, approximately one third of whom have been randomized to each of three treatment groups:

- a low dose leuprolide acetate group, in which participants will receive the same dose as the high dose group in ALADDIN I;

- a high dose leuprolide acetate group, in which participants will receive a dose equal to 150% of the high dose administered in ALADDIN I; and

- a placebo group.

Each participant will be administered two injections containing either drug or placebo every 12 weeks during the trial.

The primary efficacy endpoints in this trial are change from baseline at 48 weeks in ADAS-Cog scores and change from baseline at 48 weeks in ADCS-CGIC scores in trial participants who are also taking ACIs. Secondary efficacy endpoints include ADCS-ADL changes from baseline at week 48 in participants who are also taking ACIs.

Appendix H: Lupron-Drug Facts

Leuprolide

Clinical data

Trade names Lupron

Pharmacokinetic data

Half-life 3 hours

Excretion Renal

Chemical data

Formula $C_{59}H_{84}N_{16}O_{12}$

Mol. mass 1209.4 g/mol

Leuprorelin (INN) or **leuprolide acetate** (USAN) is a GnRH analog. Proper Sequence: Pyr-His-Trp-Ser-Tyr-D-Leu-Leu-Arg-Pro-NHEt (Pyr = L-Pyroglutamyl)

Mode of action

Leuprolide acts as an agonist at pituitary GnRH receptors. By interrupting the normal pulsatile stimulation and the desensitization of the GnRH receptors; it indirectly down regulates the secretion of gonadotropins luteinizing hormone (LH) and follicle-stimulating hormone (FSH) leading to hypo-gonadism and thus a dramatic reduction in estradiol and testosterone levels in both sexes.

Clinical use

An LH-RH (GnRH) analog, leuprolide may be used in the treatment of hormone-responsive cancers such as prostate cancer or breast cancer, estrogen-dependent conditions (such as endometrio-sis[1] or uterine fibroids), to treat precocious puberty,[2] and to control ovarian stimulation in In Vitro Fertilization (IVF). It is considered a possible treatment for paraphilias.[3]

Leuprolide has been tested as a treatment for reducing sexual urges in pedophiles and other cases of paraphilia.[4][5] High doses are sometimes used to chemically castrate sex offenders.[6]

Leuprolide is also under investigation for possible use in the treatment of mild to moderate Alzheimer's disease.[7]

Leuprolide is also used to treat chronic adrenal disease in ferrets. It also used for treatment of steroid abuse

Lupron protocol

A 2005 paper suggested leuprolide as a possible treatment for autism the hypothetical method of action being the now defunct hypothesis that autism is caused by mercury, with the additional unfounded assumption that mercury binds irreversibly to testosterone and therefore leuprolide can help cure autism by lowering the testosterone levels and thereby mercury levels. However, used on children or adolescents it could cause disastrous and irreversible damage to sexual functioning, and there is no scientifically valid or reliable research to show its effectiveness in treating autism. This use has been termed the "Lupron protocol" and Mark Geier, the proponent of the hypothesis, has frequently been barred from testifying in vaccine-autism related cases on the grounds of not being sufficiently expert in that particular issue and has had his medical license revoked. Medical experts have referred to Geier's claims as "junk science".

Approvals

- Lupron Injection (5 mg/mL for daily subcutaneous injection) was first approved by the FDA for treatment of advanced prostate cancer on April 9, 1985.
- Lupron Depot (7.5 mg/vial for monthly intramuscular depot injection) was first approved by the FDA for palliative treatment of advanced prostate cancer on January 26, 1989, and subsequently in 22.5 mg/vial and 30 mg/vial for intramuscular depot injection every 3 and 4 months, respectively. 3.75 mg/vial and 11.25 mg/vial dosage forms were subsequently approved for subcutaneous depot injection every month and every 3 months, respectively for treatment of endometriosis or fibroids. 7.5 mg/vial, 11.25 mg/vial,

and 15 mg/vial dosage forms were subsequently approved for subcutaneous depot injection for treatment of children with central precocious puberty.

- Viadur (72 mg yearly subcutaneous implant) was first approved by the FDA for palliative treatment of advanced prostate cancer on March 6, 2000. Bayer will fulfill orders until current supplies are depleted, expected by the end of April 2008

- Eligard (7.5 mg for monthly subcutaneous depot injection) was first approved by the FDA for palliative treatment of advanced prostate cancer on January 24, 2002, and subsequently in 22.5 mg, 30 mg, and 45 mg doses for subcutaneous depot injection every 3, 4, and 6 months, respectively.

- Leupromer® 7.5 (7.5 mg, One month depot for subcutaneous injection) is the second In-situ forming injectable drug in world. it use for palliative treatment of advanced prostate cancer, endometriosis and fibroids. it approved by The Ministry of Health and Medical Education Of Iran.

Leuprolide acetate is marketed by Bayer AG under the brand name **Viadur**, by Sanofi-Aventis under the brand name **Eligard**, and by TAP Pharmaceuticals (1985–2008) and Abbott Laboratories (2008-current) under the brand name **Lupron**. It is available as a slow-release implant or subcu-taneous/intramuscular injection.

In the UK and Ireland, leuprorelin is marketed by Takeda UK as **Prostap SR** (one-month injection) and **Prostap 3** (three-month injection).

Warnings

A study that found that leuprorelin is very risky, especially for men with heart problems. An AP article stated, "The hormone treatment was linked with a 96 percent higher risk of death after adjusting for other risk factors.A similar study issued in JAMA in July 2008 also found that the drug offered no life-prolonging benefits in men with advanced prostate cancer vs. men who did not take any form of hormone therapy, or conservative management. Women with endometriosis also suffer significant side effects.

In June 2009 the label was changed again to warn about "convulsion" in the post-marketing surveillance. The label shows that 98% of women had adverse events including 65% suffering headache/migraine, 31% depression, 31% insomnia, and 25% Nausea/vomiting. Many other adverse events are listed in the label. The label also notes that women with no history of depression or psychiatric illness reported suicidal ideation and attempts.

Additionally, leuprolide therapy in conjunction with radiation has been shown to result in a statistically significant shortening of the penis.[15]

Lupron Depot

All medicines may cause side effects, but many people have no, or minor, side effects. Check with your doctor if any of these most COMMON side effects persist or become bothersome when using Lupron Depot:

Breast tenderness; constipation; decreased sexual desire or ability; difficulty sleeping; hot flashes or sweating; infection (fever, chills, sore throat); nausea or vomiting; pain, redness, or swelling at the injection site.

Seek medical attention right away if any of these SEVERE side effects occur when using Lupron Depot:
Severe allergic reactions (rash; hives; itching; difficulty breathing; tightness in the chest; swelling of the mouth, face, lips, or tongue); blood in the urine; burning, numbness, tingling, or weakness; fainting; fast, slow, or irregular heartbeat; mental or mood changes (eg, anxiety, delusions, depression, nervousness); new or worsening bone pain; paralysis; seizures; severe dizziness or light-headedness; severe drowsiness; severe headache; shortness of breath; swelling of the hands, ankles, or feet; symptoms of heart attack (eg, chest, jaw, or left arm pain; numbness of an arm or leg; sudden, severe headache or vomiting; vision changes); symptoms of high blood sugar (eg, drowsiness; fast breathing; flushing; fruit-like breath odor; increased thirst, hunger, or urination); symptoms of stroke (eg, confusion, one-sided weakness, slurred speech, vision changes); trouble urinating or inability to urinate; vision changes.

Lupron Depot 11.25 mg Depot Suspension

All medicines may cause side effects, but many people have no, or minor, side effects. Check with your doctor if any of these most COMMON side effects persist or become bothersome when using Lupron Depot 11.25 mg Depot Suspension:

Acne; changes in weight; dizziness; general body pain; injection-site irritation (eg, mild burning, itching, pain, stinging, swelling); nausea or vomiting; trouble sleeping; weakness.

Seek medical attention right away if any of these SEVERE side effects occur when using Lupron Depot 11.25 mg Depot Suspension:
Severe allergic reactions (rash; hives; itching; difficulty breathing; tightness in the chest; swelling of the mouth, face, lips, or tongue); black, tarry stools; blood in the urine; burning, numbness, or tingling; decreased hearing; fainting; memory problems; new or worsening bone pain; new or worsening mood or mental changes (eg, anxiety, delusions, depression, memory problems, nervousness); paralysis; seizures; severe dizziness or light-headedness; severe drowsiness; severe headache; shortness of breath; slow, fast, or irregular heartbeat; swelling of the hands, ankles, or feet; symptoms of heart attack (eg, chest, jaw, or left arm pain; numbness of an arm or leg; sudden, severe headache or vomiting; vision changes); symptoms of high blood sugar (eg, drowsiness; fast breathing; flushing; fruit-like breath odor; increased thirst, hunger, or urination); symptoms of infection (eg, chills, fever);

symptoms of stroke (eg, confusion, one-sided weakness, slurred speech, vision changes); trouble urinating (eg, loss of bladder control, unable to urinate, painful urination); unusual vaginal itching, irritation, discharge, or odor; vision changes or blurred vision; vomit that looks like coffee grounds.

Appendix I: Pregnenolone

J Clin Endocrinol Metab. 2002 May;87(5):2225-31.

Sex- and age-related changes in epitestosterone in relation to pregnenolone sulfate and testosterone in normal subjects.

Havlíková H Hill M Hampl R Stárka L

Source

Institute of Endocrinology, CZ 116 94 Prague, Czech Republic.

Abstract
Epitestosterone has been demonstrated to act at various levels as a weak antiandrogen. So far, its serum levels have been followed up only in males. Epitestosterone and its major circulating precursor pregnenolone sulfate and T were measured in serum from 211 healthy women and 386 men to find out whether serum concentrations of epitestosterone are sufficient to exert its antiandrogenic actions. In women, epitestosterone exhibited a maximum around 20 yr of age, followed by a continuous decline up to menopause and by a further increase in the postmenopause. In men, maximum epitestosterone levels were detected at around 35 yr of age, followed by a continuous decrease. Pregnenolone sulfate levels in women reached their maximum at about age 32 yr and then declined continuously, and in males the maximum was reached about 5 yr earlier and then remained nearly constant. Epitestosterone correlated with pregnenolone sulfate only

in males. In both sexes a sharp decrease of the epitestosterone/T ratio around puberty occurred. In conclusion, concentrations of epitestosterone and pregnenolone sulfate are age dependent and, at least in prepubertal boys and girls, epitestosterone reaches or even exceeds the concentrations of T, thus supporting its role as an endogenous antiandrogen. The dissimilarities in the course of epitestosterone levels through the lifespan of men and women and its relation to pregnenolone sulfate concentrations raise the question of the contribution of the adrenals and gonads to the production of both steroids and even to the uniformity of the mechanism of epitestosterone formation.

Pregnenolone: The "Happiness" Hormone

By Steve Barwick on 11/19/2008

When Oscar-winning comedic actress Goldie Hawn was asked recently in a Vanity Faire interview, "When you were a child, what did you want to be when you grew up?" she replied with a single word: "Happy."

Most of us can relate to that simple, honest childhood desire for happiness. Unfortunately, as we grow older, a host of subtle and some not-so-subtle changes begin to take place in our bodies. And those changes can lead to a number of health challenges that can rob you of your energy, vitality, stamina, physical strength, mental acuity and yes, even your emotional well-being, i.e., your happiness.

One of the most important age-related changes for both men and women alike is the drop in your body's levels of a simple, yet profoundly important hormone called pregnenolone. Much like DHEA, pregnenolone is a completely natural hormone manufactured in the body from cholesterol. Indeed, pregnenolone is the grand precursor from which almost all of the other steroid hormones are made, including DHEA, progesterone, testosterone, the estrogens, and cortisol. This is why it is frequently referred to as the "mother hormone."

According to Dr. Joseph Mercola, DO, best-selling author of the *The Total Health Program*:

- "With both men and women alike, pregnenolone levels naturally peak during youth and begin a long, slow decline with age. By the age of 75 our bodies produce 60% less pregnenolone than the levels produced in our mid-30's. For this reason pregnenolone is one of the biomarkers of aging. Like counting the rings of a tree, by measuring the level of pregnenolone at any given point of a person's life, it is often possible to make an educated guess as to his or her age."

Indeed, many cutting edge physicians and scientists now believe that raising your body's levels of pregnenolone to more youthful levels is a crucial step in the prevention of premature aging. "If you're feeling older than your days," says well-known biologist and author Jim South, M.A., "then pregnenolone may be just what you need."

'The Happiness Hormone'

Pregnenolone has also been widely reported to make people feel happier. In fact, its well-known mood-heightening qualities are almost legendary. As Dr. Ray Sahelian, MD states in his wonderful little book, *Pregnenolone: Nature's Feel-Good Hormone:*

- "I am 100 percent convinced that taking pregnenolone leads to changes in awareness and alertness. I noticed an improved visual clarity...within an hour of dosing...a mellow, steady, persistent feeling of well-being...had imperceptibly come on...Flowers seemed...brighter and prettier...my attention focused on the architecture of the homes...I started noticing the patterns of the stones, the shapes of the windows, doorways, porticos and other details...the palm trees...appeared Caribbean island-like picturesque. Everything seemed more beautiful and intriguing. I felt a sense of child wonder, that everything was okay. How special and enchanting life could be!"

Dr. William Regelson, a respected pregnenolone expert and author of *The Superhormone Promise: Nature's Antidote to Aging*, writes that there appears to be a direct correlation between pregnenolone levels in the human body and emotional well-being. He states, "A recent study conducted by the National Institutes of Mental Health showed that people with clinical depression have lower than normal amounts of pregnenolone in their cerebral spinal fluid (the fluid that literally bathes the brain)." In other words, as pregnenolone levels decline, your emotional well-being can also sink like a stone.

Other experts point to pregnenolone's ability to help reduce excessively high levels of the stress hormone, cortisol, as the reason it has such a profoundly positive balancing effect on the emotions. According to Dr. Keith Scott-Mumby, MB ChB, MD, PhD, FRCP, MA,

- "Pregnenolone has been studied extensively since the 1940's...One of its most important actions is to counter damage caused by the natural stress hormone called 'cortisol.' Cortisol is helpful in modest amounts, but is toxic at higher levels. Pregnenolone's ability to block excess cortisol levels may be one of the main reasons for its known memory-enhancing and mood-boosting benefits."

Pregnenolone also appears to help people approach life's daily challenges with a more positive mental outlook. According to the respected biologist and author Dr. Ray

Peat, PhD, "When using pregnenolone, men and women alike report feeling a profound mood of resilience and an increased ability to confront challenges successfully."

In the book, The Mood Cure, by Julia Ross, M.A., pregnenolone supplementation is highly recommended for helping overcome adrenal fatigue and reversing even the most devastating forms of exhaustion, emotional distress and depression. And in the book, Pregnenolone: A Radical New Approach to Health, Longevity, and Emotional Well-Being, author Dr. Gary Young, N.D., points out that pregnenolone enhances mental performance, facilitates learning, helps the body adapt to stress, increases one's overall feeling of happiness and well-being, and helps induce a change of attitude in which we actually become more appreciative of life.

According to Dr. Young, pregnenolone also improves concentration, prevents mental fatigue, increases productivity, improves psychomotor performance and relieves depression. In short, restoring pregnenolone to more youthful levels in the body helps boost not only our emotional well-being, but enhances our physical and cognitive abilities as well.

Better Memory, Focus and Concentration!

Pregnenolone also operates as a powerful neurosteroid in the brain, modulating the transmission of messages from neuron to neuron, and strongly influencing learning and memory processes. In other words, it helps you think quicker, understand and retain more complex topics, and even speak with greater clarity.

In animal tests, pregnenolone has been found to be 100 times more effective for memory enhancement than any other steroid, steroid-precursor or prescription drug tested. According to the Proceedings of the National Academy of Sciences (Nov. 6, 1995), pregnenolone is "The most potent memory enhancer yet found."

In a recent Life Extension Foundation article titled "Enhancing Cognitive Function With Pregnenolone," Dr. Julius G. Goepp, MD wrote:

- "There is strong evidence that pregnenolone levels diminish with advancing age and that restoring these levels may help alleviate deteriorating brain function...This is borne out in research that has demonstrated pregnenolone's ability to reduce the risk of dementia and improve memory, while also alleviating anxiety and fighting depression...Pregnenolone may play a pivotal role both in laying down memories in the first place, and then preventing their loss by directly protecting the nerve networks that store them! These complementary and versatile actions of pregnenolone are sending shock waves of interest through the scientific community because of the enormous implications for treating all sorts of age-related disorders of memory"

Dr. Goepp also points out, "Even more remarkably, from a treatment standpoint, researchers have shown that pregnenolone increases brain levels of acetylcholine, a key neurotransmitter required for optimal brain function, which becomes deficient in patients with Alzheimer's disease. Acetylcholine is not only vital for thought and memory, it is also involved in controlling sleep cycles, especially the phase of sleep that is associated with memory (called paradoxical sleep or the random eye movement [REM] phase). Scientists have used this knowledge to study the effects of pregnenolone on sleep cycles and discovered that it dramatically increases memory-enhancing sleep. Together with previous findings that pregnenolone increases nerve cell growth (neurogenesis), researchers have concluded that pregnenolone can improve cognitive function in older animals by increasing acetylcholine levels, which stimulate new nerve cell growth in the brain areas most closely associated with memory and learning."

In clinical research pregnenolone has been demonstrated to be one of the safest and least toxic substances ever tested, with dosages in the hundreds of milligrams showing no toxicity whatsoever. While much smaller doses in the 5 mg. to 20 mg. range are widely used in nutritional supplementation programs, as with all supplements you should nevertheless tell your doctor if you are taking pregnenolone.

Additionally, men diagnosed with prostate cancer (which theoretically may be worsened by increased testosterone levels) and women with breast or ovarian cancer (which theoretically may be worsened by increased estrogen levels) should check with their doctors first before taking pregnenolone. Men with high PSA (prostate specific antigen) blood levels (possible indicator for undiagnosed or future prostate cancer) should also check with their doctors first.

What's more, because of pregnenolone's beneficial "uplifting" effects on the brain (i.e., it increases the firing of the neurons between the synapses for quicker thinking and greater clarity), people known to suffer from epileptic seizures or who are taking an anti-seizure medication such as Dilantin, Depakote or Tegretol should only use pregnenolone with their doctor's supervision.

Finally, people diagnosed with heart palpitations or arrhythmias should also check with their doctors first before using pregnenolone due to its lightly stimulating effects on the body's overall metabolism.

Appendix J: Scientists Pinpoint How Vitamin D May Help Clear Amyloid Plaques Found in Alzheimer's

Science Daily (Mar. 6, 2012) — A team of academic researchers has identified the intracellular mechanisms regulated by vitamin D3 that may help the body clear the brain of amyloid beta, the main component of plaques associated with Alzheimer's disease.

See Also:

Health & Medicine
Published in the March 6 issue of the *Journal of Alzheimer's Disease,* the early findings show that vitamin D3 may activate key genes and cellular signaling networks to help stimulate the immune system to clear the amyloid-beta protein.

Previous laboratory work by the team demonstrated that specific types of immune cells in Alzheimer's patients may respond to therapy with vitamin D3 and curcumin, a chemical found in turmeric spice, by stimulating the innate immune system to clear amyloid beta. But the researchers didn't know how it worked.

"This new study helped clarify the key mechanisms involved, which will help us better understand the usefulness of vitamin D3 and curcumin as possible therapies for Alzheimer's disease," said study author Dr. Milan Fiala, a researcher at the David Geffen School of Medicine at UCLA and the Veterans Affairs Greater Los Angeles Healthcare System.

For the study, scientists drew blood samples from Alzheimer's patients and healthy controls and then isolated critical immune cells from the blood called macrophages, which are responsible for gobbling up amyloid beta and other waste products in the brain and body.

The team incubated the immune cells overnight with amyloid beta. An active form of vitamin D3 called 1a,25-dihydroxyvitamin D3, which is made in the body by enzymatic conversion in the liver and kidneys, was added to some of the cells to gauge the effect it had on amyloid beta absorption.

Previous work by the team, based on the function of Alzheimer's patients' macrophages, showed that there are at least two types of patients and macrophages: Type I macrophages are improved by addition of 1a,25-dihydroxyvitamin D3 and curcuminoids (a synthetic form of curcumin), while Type II macrophages are improved only by adding 1a,25-dihydroxyvitamin D3.

Researchers found that in both Type I and Type II macrophages, the added 1a,25-dihydroxyvitamin D3 played a key role in opening a specific chloride channel called "chloride channel 3 (CLC3)," which is important in supporting the uptake of amyloid beta through the process known as phagocytosis. Curcuminoids activated this chloride channel only in Type I macrophages. The scientists also found that 1a,25-dihydroxyvitamin D3 strongly helped trigger the genetic transcription of the chloride channel and the receptor for 1a,25-dihydroxyvitamin D3 in Type II macrophages. Transcription is the first step leading to gene expression.

The mechanisms behind the effects of 1a,25-dihydroxyvitamin D3 on phagocytosis were complex and dependent on calcium and signaling by the "MAPK" pathway, which helps communicate a signal from the vitamin D3 receptor located on the surface of a cell to the DNA in the cell's nucleus.

The pivotal effect of 1a,25-dihydroxyvitamin D3 was shown in a collaboration between Dr. Patrick R. Griffin from the Scripps Research Institute and Dr. Mathew T. Mizwicki from UC Riverside. They utilized a technique based on mass spectrometry, which showed that 1a,25-dihydroxyvitamin D3 stabilized many more critical sites on the vitamin D receptor than did the curcuminoids.

"Our findings demonstrate that active forms of vitamin D3 may be an important regulator of immune activities of macrophages in helping to clear amyloid plaques by directly regulating the expression of genes, as well as the structural physical workings of the cells," said study author Mizwicki, who was an assistant research biochemist in the department of biochemistry at UC Riverside when the study was conducted.

According to the team, one of the next stages of research would be a clinical trial with vitamin D3 to assess the impact on Alzheimer's disease patients. Previous studies by other teams have shown that a low serum level of 25-hydroxyvitamin D3 may be associated with cognitive decline. It is too early to recommend a definitive dosage of vitamin D3 to help with Alzheimer's disease and brain health, the researchers said.

Appendix K: New Findings Contradict Dominant Theory in Alzheimer's Disease

ScienceDaily (Oct. 28, 2011) — For decades the amyloid hypothesis has dominated the research field in Alzheimer's disease. The theory describes how an increase in secreted beta-amyloid peptides leads to the formation of plaques, toxic clusters of damaged proteins between cells, which eventually result in neurodegeneration. Scientists at Lund University, Sweden, have now presented a study that turns this premise on its head. The research group's data offers an opposite hypothesis, suggesting that it is in fact the neurons' inability to secrete beta-amyloid that is at the heart of pathogenesis in Alzheimer's disease.

The study, published in the October issue of the *Journal of Neuroscience*, shows an increase in unwanted *intracellular* beta-amyloid occurring early on in Alzheimer's disease. The accumulation of beta-amyloid inside the neuron is here shown to be caused by the loss of normal function to secrete beta-amyloid.

Contrary to the dominant theory, where aggregated extracellular beta-amyloid is considered the main culprit, the study instead demonstrates that reduced secretion of beta-amyloid signals the beginning of the disease.

The damage to the neuron, created by the aggregated toxic beta-amyloid *inside* the cell, is believed to be a prior step to the formation of plaques, the long-time hallmark biomarker of the disease.

Professor Gunnar Gouras, the senior researcher of the study, hopes that the surprising new findings can help push the research field in a new direction.

"The many investigators and pharmaceutical companies screening for compounds that reduce secreted beta-amyloid have it the *wrong way around*. The problem is rather *the opposite*, that it is *not* getting secreted. To find the root of the disease, we now need to focus on this critical intracellular pool of beta-amyloid.

"We are showing here that the increase of intracellular beta-amyloid is one of the earliest events occurring in Alzheimer's disease, before the formation of plaques. Our experiments clearly show a decreased secretion of beta-amyloid in our primary neuron disease model. This is probably because the cell's metabolism and secretion pathways are disrupted in some way, leading beta-amyloid to be accumulated inside the cell instead of being secreted naturally," says David
Tampellini, first author of the study.

The theory of early accumulation of beta-amyloid inside the cell offers an alternate explanation for the formation of plaques. When excess amounts of beta-amyloid start to build up inside the cell, it is also stored in synapses. When the synapses can no longer hold the increasing amounts of the toxic peptide the membrane breaks, releasing the waste into the extracellular space. The toxins released now create the seed for other amyloids to gather and start forming the plaques.

Book Overview

Tired of Big Pharma Alzheimer's treatments that do *not* work? Tried Aricept, Namenda, Razadyne, Exelon, Cognex, all to no avail?

It's time to take control of your Alzheimer's treatment, and try protocols that have actually *worked*, based on the newest, latest, cutting-edge, correct theory.

The latest theory is that Alzheimer's is caused by the huge increase in the reproduction-related hormone--*Luteinizing Hormone* (LH)--that occurs in both men and women after age 50 (up to 1,000's of %). Just like annual plants and Pacific Salmon that are killed after a burst of reproduction by their reproductive hormones--humans undergo the same process, except in slow motion. LH is literally eating away at our brains and bodies.

The evidence that the "LH causes AD" theory is true is becoming larger and even attracting scientists from the ultra-conservative NIH (National Institutes of Health). It is all detailed here in this book.

When the hormone LH rises too much in young children, it causes precocious puberty (reaching sexual maturity as young as 5 years old). To stop precocious puberty, doctors have been using Lupron injections for years, which stops the rise in LH.

Lupron injections have also been used successfully to STOP the progression of Alzheimer's in a small pilot study, which is described in detail in this book.

Melatonin, which also suppresses LH has also been shown to STOP the progression of AD. The melatonin study is also described in detail in this book.

Why doesn't Big Pharma promote new treatments based on this cutting edge new theory--BECAUSE THEY CAN'T MAKE ANY MONEY ON IT. They would rather keep selling you Aricept and pretending they don't accept the new evidence. Heck--they probably think you are eventually going to die anyway, so what's the big deal?

Anyone can buy melatonin over the counter, and any doctor can write a prescription for Lupron, which is about to go off patent in 2015!

Read this book and follow its protocols to stop Alzheimer's in its tracks.

Also, learn about the fantastic promise of high dose-melatonin as a treatment for AD and possible side effects to look out for, based on my year-long experiment and the experience of my friends taking huge doses of melatonin. This is by far your best chance at stopping Alzheimer's.

About The Author

This IS the better mousetrap! Most MD's get just a basic 4 years in Med School, then work to earn, not learn. I've researched diseases and aging for 20+ years, with a 10 year stint where I spent 12 hrs/day everyday in the Northwestern Med School's library reviewing clinical and scientific studies. I've had 3 major papers published; the journal that published my articles has 5 Nobel Prizes between the editors, and described my papers as *"extremely exciting and of major importance."*